ABC of
Complementary Medicine

Second Edition

ABC series

The revised and updated ABC series – written by specialists for non-specialists

- With over 40 titles, this extensive series provides a quick and dependable reference on a broad range of topics in all the major specialities

- An easy-to-use resource, covering the symptoms, investigations, treatment and management of conditions presenting in your day-to-day practice

- Full colour photographs and illustrations aid diagnosis and patient understanding of a condition

- Each book in the new series now offers links to further information and articles, and a new dedicated website provides even more support

- A highly illustrated, informative and practical source of knowledge for GPs, GP registrars, junior doctors, doctors in training and those in primary care

For further information on the entire ABC series, please visit:

www.abcbookseries.com

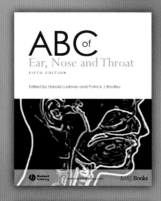

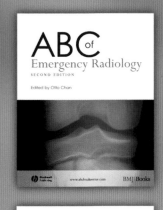

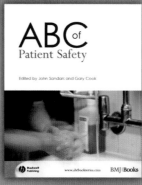

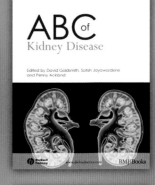

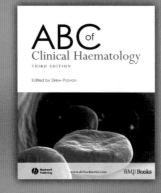

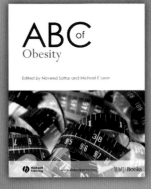

WILEY-BLACKWELL

BMJ | Books

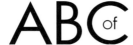

ABC of

Complementary
Medicine

Second Edition

EDITED BY

Catherine Zollman

General Practitioner
Bristol, UK

Andrew Vickers

Associate Attending Research Methodologist
Department of Epidemiology and Biostatistics, Memorial Sloan-Kettering Cancer Center
New York, USA

Janet Richardson

Professor of Health Service Research
Faculty of Health and Social Work, University of Plymouth
Plymouth, UK

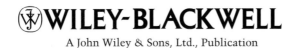

A John Wiley & Sons, Ltd., Publication

BMJ|Books

Library of Congress Cataloguing-in-Publication Data

Zollman, Catherine.
    ABC of complementary medicine / Catherine Zollman, Andrew Vickers, Janet Richardson -- 2nd ed.
        p. ; cm.
    Includes bibliographical references and index.
    ISBN-13: 978-1-4051-3657-0 (alk. paper)
    ISBN-10: 1-4051-3657-X (alk. paper)
    1. Alternative medicine. I. Richardson, Janet, Dr. II. Vickers, Andrew. III. Title.
    [DNLM: 1. Complementary Therapies. WB 890 Z86a 2008]
    R733.Z65 2008
    610--dc22

                                                                    2007038357

ISBN: 978-1-4051-3657-0

A catalogue record for this book is available from the British Library.

Set in 9.25/12 pt Minion by Newgen Imaging Systems Pvt. Ltd, Chennai, India
Printed in Singapore by Utopia Press Pte Ltd

1 2008

Contents

Contributors

Alan Breen

Professor, IMRCI-Anglo-European College of Chiropractic, Bournemouth, UK

Ian Brownhill

Programmes Director, The Prince's Foundation for Integrated Health, London, UK

Sheila Dane

Development Officer, Partnership and Forums, Kensington and Chelsea Social Council, London, UK

Eleanor Lines

Publishing Consultant in Complementary Medicine and Commissioning Editor, iCAM Newsletter, University of Westminster, London, UK

Gillian McCall

Specialist Radiographer, Department of Clinical Oncology, St Thomas' Hospital, London, UK

Amanda Nadin

Development Manager, iCAM, School of Integrated Health, University of Westminster, London, UK

Kate Neil

Managing Director, Centre for Nutrition Education, Wokingham, UK

Clare Relton

Research Associate, School of Health and Related Research, University of Sheffield, Sheffield, UK

Janet Richardson

Professor of Health Service Research, Faculty of Health and Social Work, University of Plymouth, Plymouth, UK

Kate Thomas

Professor, Complementary and Alternative Medicine Research, School of Healthcare, University of Leeds, Leeds, UK

Andrew Vickers

Associate Attending Research Methodologist, Department of Epidemiology and Biostatistics, Memorial Sloan-Kettering Cancer Center, New York, USA

Jane Wilkinson

Director, iCAM, School of Integrated Health, University of Westminster, London, UK

Catherine Zollman

General Practitioner, Bristol, UK

CHAPTER 1

What is Complementary Medicine?

Catherine Zollman

Definitions and terms

Complementary medicine refers to a group of therapeutic and diagnostic disciplines that exist largely outside the institutions where conventional health care is taught and provided. Complementary medicine is an increasing feature of healthcare practice, but considerable confusion remains about what exactly it is and what position the disciplines included under this term should hold in relation to conventional medicine.

In the 1970s and 1980s these disciplines were mainly provided as an alternative to conventional health care and hence became known collectively as 'alternative medicine'. The name 'complementary medicine' developed as the two systems began to be used alongside (to 'complement') each other. Over the years, 'complementary' has changed from describing this relationship between unconventional healthcare disciplines and conventional care to defining the group of disciplines itself. Some authorities use the term 'unconventional medicine' synonymously. More recently the terms 'integrative' and 'integrated' medicine have been used to describe the delivery of complementary therapies within conventional healthcare settings. This changing and overlapping terminology may explain some of the confusion that surrounds the subject.

We use the term complementary medicine to describe healthcare practices such as those listed in Box 1.1. We use it synonymously with the terms 'complementary therapies' and 'complementary and alternative medicine' found in other texts, according to the definition used by the Cochrane Collaboration.

Which disciplines are complementary?

Our list is not exhaustive, and new branches of established disciplines are continually being developed. Also, what is thought to be conventional varies between countries and changes over time. The boundary between complementary and conventional medicine is therefore blurred and constantly shifting. For example, although osteopathy and chiropractic are still predominantly practised outside the NHS in Britain, they are subject to statutory regulation and included as part of standard care in guidelines from conventional bodies such as the Royal College of General Practitioners.

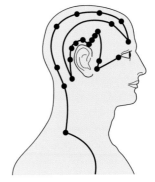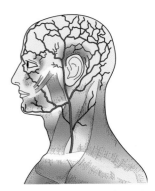

Figure 1.1 Some important superficial features of the head and neck from an acupuncture and a conventional medical perspective.

Box 1.1 **Common complementary therapies**

- Acupressure
- Acupuncture*
- Alexander technique
- Anthroposophic medicine
- Applied kinesiology
- Aromatherapy*
- Autogenic training
- Ayurveda
- Chiropractic*
- Cranial osteopathy
- Environmental medicine
- Healing*
- Herbal medicine*
- Homeopathy*
- Hypnosis*
- Massage*
- Meditation*
- Naturopathy
- Nutritional therapy*
- Osteopathy*
- Reflexology*
- Reiki
- Relaxation and visualization*
- Shiatsu
- Therapeutic touch
- Yoga*

*Considered in detail in later chapters.

Box 1.2 **Definition of complementary medicine adopted by the Cochrane Collaboration Complementary Medicine Field**

Complementary medicine includes all such practices and ideas which are outside the domain of conventional medicine in several countries and defined by their users as preventing or treating illness, or promoting health and well being. These practices complement mainstream medicine by (1) contributing to a common whole, (2) satisfying a demand not met by conventional practices, and (3) diversifying the conceptual framework of medicine.

The wide range of disciplines classified as complementary medicine makes it difficult to find defining criteria that are common to all. Many of the assumptions made about complementary medicine are oversimplistic generalizations.

Organizational structure

Historical development

Since the inception of the NHS, the public sector has supported training, regulation, research, and practice in conventional health care. The development of complementary medicine has taken place largely in the private sector. Until recently, most complementary practitioners trained in small, privately funded colleges and then worked independently in relative isolation from other practitioners. An increasing number of complementary therapies are now taught at degree and masters level in universities.

Research

More complementary medical research exists than is commonly recognized – the Cochrane Library lists over 6000 randomized trials and around 150 Cochrane reviews of complementary and alternative medicine (CAM) have been published, but the field is still poorly researched compared with conventional medicine. There are several reasons for this, some of which also apply to conventional disciplines like surgery, occupational therapy, and speech therapy (see Box 1.4). However, complementary practitioners are increasingly aware of the value of research, and many complementary therapy training courses now include research skills. Conventional sources of funding, such as the NHS research and development programme and major cancer charities, have become more open to complementary researchers. Programmes to build the capacity for research into complementary therapies have been introduced into several UK universities as a result of recommendations in the House of Lords Report, 2000. However funding for research in complementary medicine is still relatively small scale.

Training

Although complementary practitioners (other than osteopaths and chiropractors) can legally practise without any training whatsoever, most have completed some further education in their chosen discipline.

There is great variation in the many training institutions. For the major therapies – osteopathy, chiropractic, acupuncture, herbal medicine, and homeopathy – these tend to be highly developed. Some are delivered within universities, with degree level exams and external assessment. Others, particularly those teaching less invasive therapies such as reflexology and aromatherapy, tend to be small and isolated schools that determine curricula internally and have idiosyncratic assessment procedures. In some courses direct clinical contact is limited. Some are not recognized by the main registering bodies in the relevant discipline. Most complementary practitioners finance their training without state support (unless they are training within a university at undergraduate level), and many train part time over several years. National occupational standards (NOSs), which set competence expectations for

---

Box 1.3 **Unhelpful assumptions about complementary medicine**

Non-statutory – not provided by the NHS
- Complementary medicine is increasingly available on the NHS
- Over 40% of Primary Care Trusts (PCTs) provide access to complementary medicine for NHS patients
- Most cancer centres in the UK offer some form of complementary medicine

Unregulated – therapists not regulated by state legislation
- Osteopaths and chiropractors are state registered and regulated and other disciplines are working towards statutory regulation and have well-established voluntary self-regulation
- A substantial amount of complementary medicine is delivered by conventional health professionals

Unconventional – not taught in medical schools
- Disciplines such as nursing, physiotherapy, and chiropody are also not taught in medical schools
- A large number of complementary therapies are taught in healthcare faculties within universities
- Some medical schools have a complementary medicine component as part of the curriculum

Natural
- Good conventional medicine also involves rehabilitation with, say, rest, exercise, or diet
- Complementary medicine may involve unnatural practices such as injecting mistletoe extract or inserting needles into the skin

Holistic – treats the whole person
- Many conventional healthcare professionals work in a holistic manner
- Complementary therapists can be narrow and reductionist in their approach
- Holism relates more to the outlook of the practitioner than to the type of medicine practised

Alternative
- Implies use instead of conventional treatment
- Most users of complementary medicine seem not to have abandoned conventional medicine

Unproved
- There is a growing body of evidence that certain complementary therapies are effective in certain clinical conditions
- Many conventional healthcare practices are not supported by the results of controlled clinical trials

Irrational – no scientific basis
- Scientific research is starting to uncover the mechanisms of some complementary therapies, such as acupuncture and hypnosis

Harmless
- There are reports of serious adverse effects associated with using complementary medicine
- Adverse effects may be due to the specific therapy (for example a herbal product), to a non-specific effect of using complementary medicine (such as stopping a beneficial conventional medication), to an interaction with another treatment, or to the competence of the practitioner

Box 1.4 **Factors limiting research in complementary medicine**

- *Lack of research skills* – complementary practitioners have traditionally had no training in critical evaluation of existing research or practical research skills. However, research now features on some training programmes and a number of practitioners now study to masters and PhD level
- *Lack of an academic infrastructure* – most CAM practitioners have limited access to computer and library facilities, statistical support, academic supervision, and university research grants. However, a number of academic centres of excellence in CAM research are developing and this will support research capacity in CAM
- *Insufficient patient numbers* – individual list sizes are small, and most practitioners have no disease 'specialty' and therefore see very small numbers of patients with the same clinical condition. Recruiting patients into studies is difficult in private practice
- *Difficulty undertaking and interpreting systematic reviews* – poor quality studies make interpretation of results difficult. Many different types of treatment exist within each complementary discipline (for example, formula, individualized, electro, laser, and auricular acupuncture)
- *Methodological issues* – responses to treatment are unpredictable and individual, and treatment is usually not standardized. Designing appropriate controls for some complementary therapies (such as acupuncture or manipulation) is difficult, as is blinding patients to treatment allocation. Allowing for the role of the therapeutic relationship also creates problems

Box 1.5 **Complementary medicine professions working towards self-regulation**

Professions working towards statutory self-regulation
There is no single governing body but working parties with representatives from a range of regulatory organizations report to the Department of Health.
- Acupuncture: Acupuncture Stakeholders Group
- Herbal medicine: Herbal Medicine Working Group
- Chinese medicine: Chinese Medicine Working Group

Professions working towards voluntary self-regulation by a single governing body
- Alexander technique: Alexander Technique Voluntary Self Regulation Group
- Aromatherapy: Aromatherapy Consortium
- Bowen therapy: Bowen Forum
- Craniosacral therapy: Cranial Forum
- Homeopathy:* Council of Organisations Registering Homeopaths
- Massage therapy: General Council for Massage Therapy
- Nutritional therapy: Nutritional Therapy Council
- Reflexology: Reflexology Forum
- Reiki: Reiki Regulatory Working Group
- Shiatsu: General Shiatsu Council
- Spiritual healing: UK Healers
- Yoga therapy: British Council for Yoga Therapy

*Statutorily regulated health professionals who also practice homeopathy may become members of the Faculty of Homeopathy.
Modified from Prince of Wales's Foundation for Integrated Healthcare (2005).

state-run courses, describe best practice (and are used in training and recruitment). NOSs have already been published for aromatherapy, herbal medicine, homeopathy, hypnotherapy, kinesiology, reflexology, nutritional therapy, and therapeutic massage, with draft standards available for Alexander technique, spiritual healing, acupuncture, and reiki. Standards for Bowen technique, craniosacral therapy, and yoga therapy are in development.

Conventional healthcare practitioners such as nurses and doctors have their own separate training courses in some disciplines, including homeopathy and acupuncture.

Regulation

Apart from osteopaths and chiropractors, complementary practitioners are not obliged to join any official register before setting up in practice. However, many practitioners are now members of appropriate registering or accrediting bodies. There are between 150 and 300 such organizations, with varying membership size and professional standards. Some complementary disciplines may have as many as 50 registering organizations, all with different criteria and standards.

Recognizing that this situation is unsatisfactory, many disciplines are taking steps to become unified under one regulatory body per discipline. Such bodies should, as a minimum, have published criteria for entry, established codes of conduct, complaints procedures, and disciplinary sanctions, and should require members to be fully insured. The Prince of Wales's Foundation for Integrated Healthcare is working with a number of comple-

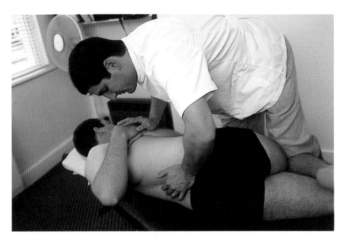

Figure 1.2 The General Osteopathic Council and General Chiropractic Council have been established by Acts of Parliament to regulate their respective disciplines. Reproduced with permission of BMJ/Ulrike Preuss.

mentary healthcare professions who are developing voluntary self-regulatory structures. The work is funded by the Department of Health.

The General Osteopathic Council and General Chiropractic Council have been established by Acts of Parliament and have statutory self-regulatory status and similar powers and functions to those of the General Medical Council. The government has established a joint working party for acupuncture and herbal medicine to progress joint statutory regulation of these professions.

Efficient regulation of the 'less invasive' complementary therapies such as massage or relaxation therapies is also important. However, statutory regulation, with its requirements for parliamentary legislation and expensive bureaucratic procedures, may not be feasible. Legal and ethics experts argue that unified and efficient voluntary self-regulatory bodies that fulfil the minimum standards listed above should be sufficient to safeguard patients. Many disciplines have established, or are working towards, a single regulatory body. It will be some years before even this is achieved across the board. Conventional healthcare professionals practising CAM should either be registered and regulated by one of the CAM regulatory bodies, or, if they are practising under their own professional regulations ('primary regulator'), 'the government has recommended that each statutory health regulator, whose members make significant use of complementary medicine, should develop clear guidelines for members on both competencies and training required for the safe and effective practice of the leading complementary disciplines'.

Approaches to treatment

The approaches used by different complementary practitioners have some common features. Although they are not shared by all complementary disciplines, and some apply to conventional disciplines as well, understanding them may help to make sense of patients' experiences of complementary medicine.

Holistic approach

Many, but not all, complementary practitioners have a multifactorial and multilevel view of human illness. Disease is thought to result from disturbances at a combination of physical,

---

Box 1.6 **Example of a holistic approach: Rudolph Steiner's central tenets of anthroposophy**

- Each individual is unique
- Scientific, artistic, and spiritual insights may need to be applied together to restore health
- Life has meaning and purpose – the loss of this sense may lead to a deterioration in health
- Illness may provide opportunities for positive change and a new balance in our lives

---

psychological, social, and spiritual levels. The body's capacity for self-repair, given appropriate conditions, is emphasized.

According to most complementary practitioners, the purpose of therapeutic intervention is to restore balance and facilitate the body's own healing responses rather than to target individual disease processes or stop troublesome symptoms. They may therefore prescribe a package of care, which could include modification of lifestyle, dietary change, and exercise as well as a specific treatment.

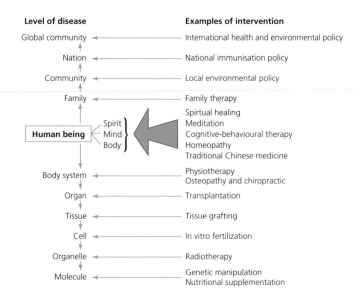

Figure 1.3 There are multiple levels of disease and, therefore, multiple levels at which therapeutic interventions can be made.

Thus, a medical herbalist may give counselling, an exercise regimen, guidance on breathing and relaxation, dietary advice, and a herbal prescription.

It should be stressed that this holistic approach is not unique to complementary practice. Good conventional general practice follows similar principles.

Use of unfamiliar terms and ideas

Complementary practitioners often use terms and ideas that are not easily translated into Western scientific language. For example, neither the reflex zones manipulated in reflexology nor the 'Qi energy' fundamental to traditional Chinese medicine have any known anatomical or physiological correlates.

Sometimes familiar terms are used but with a different meaning: acupuncturists may talk of 'taking the pulse', but they will be assessing characteristics such as 'wiriness' or 'slipperiness' which

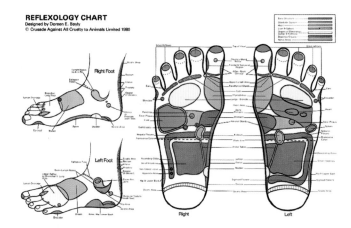

Figure 1.4 In reflexology, areas of the foot are believed to correspond to the organs or structures of the body. Reproduced with permission of the International Institute of Reflexology and the Crusade Against All Cruelty to Animals.

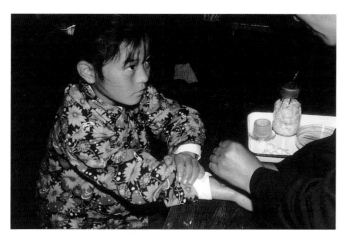

Figure 1.5 Acupuncturists may 'take a patient's pulse', but they assess characteristics such as 'wiriness' or 'slipperiness'. Reproduced with permission of Rex/SIPA Press.

have no Western equivalent. It is important not to interpret terms used in complementary medicine too literally and to understand that they are sometimes used metaphorically or as a shorthand for signs, symptoms, and syndromes that are not recognized in conventional medicine.

Different categorization of illness

Complementary and conventional practitioners often have very different methods of assessing and diagnosing patients. Thus, a patient's condition may be described as 'deficient liver Qi' by a traditional acupuncturist, as a 'pulsatilla constitution' by a homeopath, and as a 'peptic ulcer' by a conventional doctor. In each case the way the problem is diagnosed determines the treatment given.

Confusingly, there is little correlation between the different diagnostic systems: some patients with deficient liver Qi do not have ulcers, and some ulcer patients do not have deficient liver Qi but another traditional Chinese diagnosis. This causes problems when comparing complementary and conventional treatments in defined patient groups.

It should be stressed that the lack of a shared world view is not necessarily a barrier to effective cooperation. For example, doctors work closely alongside hospital chaplains and social workers, each regarding the others as valued members of the healthcare team.

Approaches to learning and teaching

Teaching and learning approaches depend to some extent on the nature of the therapy and where the therapy is taught. Where training is taken at degree level, courses include basic biological sciences, ethics, research, and reflective practice.

However, for specific therapies, their knowledge base is often derived from a tradition of clinical observation and the treatment decisions are usually empirical. Sometimes traditional teachings are handed down in a way that discourages questioning and evolution of practice, or encourages a reliance on the practitioner's own and others' individual anecdotal clinical and intuitive experiences. Where an evidence base exists, it is now much more likely to be

referred to in training and, increasingly, critical appraisal of the research literature is encouraged.

Conclusion

It is obvious from this discussion that complementary medicine is a heterogeneous subject. It is unlikely that all complementary disciplines will have an equal impact on UK health practices.

The individual complementary therapies with the most immediate relevance to the conventional healthcare professions are reviewed in detail in later chapters, but some disciplines are

> **Box 1.7 Sources of further information**
>
> - National Library for Health Complementary and Alternative Medicine Specialist Library
>   URL: http://www.library.nhs.uk/cam
> - Cochrane Complementary Medicine Field
>   URL: http://www.compmed.umm.edu/cochrane_reviews.asp#prot
> - Research Council for Complementary Medicine
>   URL: http://www.rccm.org.uk
> - Department of Health
>   URL:http://www.dh.gov.uk/en/PolicyAndGuidance/HealthAndSocial-CareTopics/ComplementaryAndAlternativeMedicine/index.htm
> - National Centre for Alternative and Complementary Medicine (US)
>   URL: http://nccam.nih.gov

inevitably beyond the scope of this book; interested readers should consult the texts and sources of information listed above.

Further reading

Berman B. Complementary medicine and medical education: teaching complementary medicine offers a way of making teaching more holistic (editorial). *BMJ* 2001; **322**: 121–2.

Ernst E. *Complementary Medicine: a critical appraisal.* Oxford: Butterworth-Heinemann, 1996.

Ernst E, Pittler M, Wider B, eds. *The Desktop Guide to Complementary and Alternative Medicine: an evidence-based approach.* St Louis: Mosby, 2005.

House of Lords Select Committee on Science and Technology, Complementary and Alternative Medicine. *HL Paper 123, Session 1999–2000.* London: HM Stationery Office, 2000.

Lewith G, Kenyon, Lewis P. *Complementary Medicine: an integrated approach.* Oxford General Practice Series. Oxford: Oxford University Press, 1996.

Mason S, Tovey P, Long AF. Evaluating complementary medicine: methodological challenges of randomised controlled trials. *BMJ* 2002; **325**: 832–4.

Mills SY. Regulation in complementary and alternative medicine. *BMJ* 2001; **322**: 158–60.

Owen DK, Lewith G, Stephens CR, Bryden H. Can doctors respond to patients' increasing interest in complementary and alternative medicine? Commentary: Special study modules and complementary and alternative medicine – the Glasgow experience. *BMJ* 2001; **322**: 154–8.

Prince of Wales's Foundation for Integrated Healthcare. *A Healthy Partnership: integrating complementary healthcare into primary care.* London: Prince of Wales's Foundation for Integrated Healthcare, 2005.

Rees L, Weil A. Integrated medicine. *BMJ* 2001; **322**: 119–20.

Spence JW, Jacobs JJ. *Complementary and Alternative Medicine: an evidence-based approach.* St Louis: Mosby, 2003.

Thomas, KJ, Coleman P, Nicholl JP. Trends in access to complementary and alternative medicines via primary care in England: 1995–2001. Results from a follow-up national survey. *Family Practice* 2003; **20**: 575–7.

Vickers A, ed. *Examining Complementary Medicine.* Cheltenham: Stanley Thomes, 1998.

Vickers A. Recent advances: complementary medicine. *BMJ* 2000; **321**: 683–6.

Vincent C, Fumham A. *Complementary Medicine: a research perspective.* London: John Wiley & Sons, Ltd, 1997.

Woodham A, Peters D. *An Encyclopaedia of Complementary Medicine.* London: Dorling Kindersley, 1997.

Yuan CS, Bieber E, Bauer BA. *Textbook of Complementary and Alternative Medicine*, 2nd edn. London: Informa Healthcare, 2006.

CHAPTER 2

Users and Practitioners of Complementary Medicine

Catherine Zollman, Kate Thomas, and Clare Relton

Complementary medicine has become more popular in Britain. Media coverage, specialist publications, and numbers of complementary therapists have all increased dramatically in the past 30 years. In this chapter we analyse this phenomenon and review available evidence about the use of complementary medicine.

Surveys of use

Several surveys, of varying quality, have been undertaken, but interpretation is often not straightforward for a number of reasons, some of which are discussed here. Some surveys target practitioners, whereas others survey patients and consumers. Different definitions of complementary medicine have been used: some include only patients consulting one of five named types of complementary practitioner, while some include up to 14 different therapies, and others include complementary medicines bought over the counter. When treatments such as hypnosis are given by conventional doctors or within conventional health services, patients and surveys may not register them as 'complementary'. However, it is possible to make estimates from the available data, which help to chart the development of complementary practice.

Levels of use

How many people use complementary medicine?

The most rigorous UK survey of the use of complementary medicine estimated that, in 1998, 46% of the population had used some form of complementary medicine. A later study estimated that in 2001 over 10% of the population had consulted a complementary practitioner in the previous year. Surveys of patients with chronic and difficult to manage diseases – such as HIV infection, multiple sclerosis, psoriasis, and rheumatological conditions – give levels of use up to twice as high. It has been estimated that in the UK one-third of patients with cancer use complementary therapies at some stage of their illness. Comparisons can be made with figures from other countries, although variations may be partly due to differences in survey methodology.

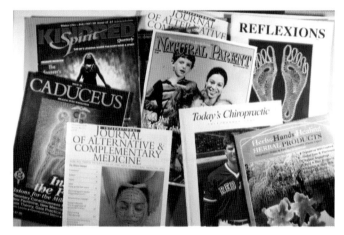

Figure 2.1 The numbers of specialist publications for complementary medicine are growing.

Table 2.1 Use of complementary medicine in UK surveys.

Survey	% of sample using complementary medicine		No. of types of therapy surveyed
	Ever used	In past year	
RSGB 1984	30%*	No data	14
Gallup 1986	14%	No data	6
Which? 1986	No data	14%	5
MORI 1989	27%*	No data	13
Thomas 1993	16.9% (33%*)	10.5%	6‡
Thomas 1998†	28.3% (46.6%*)	10.6% (28.3%*)	6

Data from Sharma (1995) and Thomas *et al.* (2001).

RSGB, Research Surveys of Great Britain.

*Includes over the counter medicines.

†Most rigorous study to date.

‡Plus 'Other complementary medicine practitioner'.

How extensively is complementary medicine used?

Attempts have been made to estimate the number of complementary medicine consultations taking place in the UK. In 1998 there

Table 2.2 Use of complementary medicine worldwide.

Country	% of sample using complementary medicine	
	Seeing a practitioner	Using any form of treatment
United Kingdom	10.5% in past year	33% ever
Australia	20% in past year	46% in past year
United States	11% in past year	34% in past year
Belgium	24% in past year	66–75% ever
France	No data	49% ever
Netherlands	6–7% in past year	18% ever
West Germany	5–12% in past year	20–30% ever

Data from surveys done during 1987–96.

Table 2.4 Popularity of different complementary therapies among users in Europe.

	% of sample using each therapy			
	Belgium	Denmark	France	Netherlands
Acupuncture	19	12	21	16
Homeopathy	56	28	32	31
Manipulation	19	23	7	No data
Herbalism	31	No data	12	No data
Reflexology	No data	39	No data	No data

Data from Fisher (1994).

were about 22 million adult consultations in the six major complementary disciplines. Average consultation rates were 4.5 per patient. An estimated 10% of consultations were provided by the NHS.

Which therapies are used?

The media often emphasize the more unusual and controversial therapies, but surveys show that most use of complementary therapy is confined to a few major disciplines. Osteopathy, chiropractic, homeopathy, acupuncture, massage, aromatherapy, and reflexology are among the most popular in the UK. Herbalism, spiritual healing, hypnotherapy, and other hands-on therapies such as shiatsu are also often mentioned. These figures mask variations in the use of individual complementary therapies among various subsections of the population. For example men are more likely to consult osteopaths and chiropractors.

The popularity of different complementary therapies varies considerably across Europe. This reflects differences in medical culture and in the historical, political, and legal position of complementary medicine in these countries.

Reasons for use

There are many myths and stereotypes about people who turn to complementary medicine – for example, that they have an

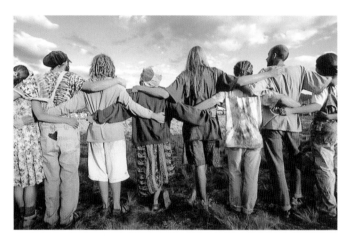

Figure 2.2 Stereotypes about the use of complementary medicine being associated with alternative lifestyles are not supported by the research evidence. Reproduced with permission of Morvan/Rex Features/SIPA Press.

alternative world view which rejects conventional medicine on principle, or that they are lured by exaggerated advertising claims. The research evidence challenges such theories.

Qualitative and quantitative studies show that people who consult complementary practitioners usually have longstanding conditions for which conventional medicine has not provided a satisfactory solution, either because it is insufficiently effective or

Table 2.3 The five most popular complementary disciplines given in five UK surveys.

RSGB 1984	*Which?* 1986	MORI 1989*†	Thomas 1993†	Thomas 1998
Acupuncture	Acupuncture	Acupuncture	Acupuncture	Osteopathy
Chiropractic	Chiropractic	Chiropractic	Chiropractic	Chiropractic
Herbal medicine‡	Herbalism	Faith healing	Herbalism	Acupuncture
Homeopathy	Homeopathy	Homeopathy	Homeopathy	Reflexology
Osteopathy	Osteopathy	Osteopathy	Osteopathy	Homeopathy

Data from Sharma (1995) and Research Council for Complementary Medicine (1998).

RSGB, Research Surveys of Great Britain.

*Did not include herbalism.

†Asked about consultations with complementary practitioners only.

‡Included over the counter products.

because it causes adverse effects. They have generally already consulted a conventional healthcare practitioner for the problem, and many continue to use the two systems concurrently. Some 'pick and mix' between complementary and conventional care, claiming that there are certain problems for which their general practitioner has the best approach and others for which a complementary practitioner is more appropriate. Most find their complementary practitioners through personal recommendation.

Once complementary therapy is started, patients' ongoing use can be broadly classified into four categories: earnest seekers, stable users, eclectic users, and one-off users. Decisions about using complementary medicine are often complex and reflect different and overlapping concerns. It is too early to assess whether the increasing availability of complementary medicine on the NHS is changing either the types of people who use complementary medicine or their reasons for doing so.

Box 2.1 **Recognized patterns of use of complementary medicine**

- *Earnest seekers* – have an intractable health problem for which they try many different forms of treatment
- *Stable users* – either use one type of therapy for most of their healthcare problems or have one main problem for which they use a regular package of one or more complementary therapies
- *Eclectic users* – choose and use different forms of therapy depending on individual problems and circumstances
- *One-off users* – discontinue complementary treatment after limited experimentation

Modified from Sharma (1995).

Who uses complementary medicine?

Survey data give us some idea of the characteristics of complementary medicine users in the United Kingdom:

- Recent evidence suggests that men and women consult complementary practitioners in equal proportion in the UK. The highest users are those aged 25–54 years (compared to users of conventional healthcare services who tend to be the very old and the very young). Children make up a relatively small proportion of users of complementary medicine, but individual therapies differ: nearly a third of the patients of some homeopaths are aged under 14, whereas acupuncturists, herbalists, and chiropractors see comparatively few children.
- Users of complementary medicine, particularly those consulting a practitioner rather than self-treating, tend to be in higher socioeconomic groups and have higher levels of education than users of conventional care.
- There has been little research into how ethnicity influences the use of complementary medicine in Britain.
- More people use complementary medicine in the south of England than in Wales, Scotland, and the north of England, but evidence suggests that this reflects access to and availability of complementary practitioners rather than to any fundamental regional differences in public attitudes or interest.

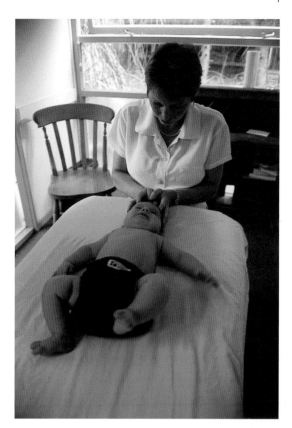

Figure 2.3 Child receiving cranial osteopathy. Reproduced with permission of BMJ/Ulrike Preuss.

Are users psychologically distinct?

Some surveys have found greater psychological morbidity, and more scepticism and negative experiences with conventional medicine, among users of complementary medicine compared with users of conventional medicine. These are not necessarily inherent differences and probably reflect the fact that most people who turn to complementary medicine do so for difficult, persisting problems that have not responded to conventional treatments.

Some heterogeneity between the users of different therapies has been identified – for example, acupuncture patients tend to have the most chronic medical histories and to be the least satisfied with their conventional treatment and general practitioner.

What conditions are treated?

In the private sector, consumer preferences indicate that the most common conditions for which patients seek complementary therapy are musculoskeletal problems, back and/or neck pain, bowel problems, indigestion, stress, anxiety, depression, migraine, and asthma. Others have problems that are not easy to categorize conventionally, such as lack of energy, and some have no specific problems but want to maintain a level of general 'wellness'. Case mix varies by therapy; for example, homeopaths and herbalists tend to treat conditions such as eczema, menstrual problems, and headaches more often than musculoskeletal problems.

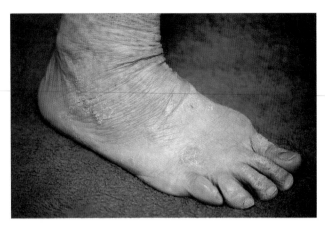

Figure 2.4 Patients are more likely to turn to complementary medicine if they have chronic, relapsing, and remitting conditions such as eczema. Reproduced with permission of BMJ/Ulrike Preuss.

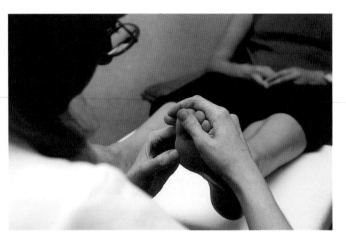

Figure 2.5 A fifth of all UK general practices provide some complementary medicine via a member of the primary healthcare team. Reproduced with permission of BMJ/Ulrike Preuss.

Complementary practitioners

The number and profile of complementary practitioners is changing rapidly. In 1981 about 13 500 registered practitioners were working in the UK. By 2000 this figure had quadrupled to about 60 000, with three disciplines – healing, aromatherapy, and reflexology – accounting for over half of all registered complementary practitioners. Although membership of these disciplines is high compared with other complementary disciplines, very few practise full time.

Nearly 10 000 conventional healthcare professionals also practise complementary medicine and are members of their own register (such as the British Medical Acupuncture Society for doctors and dentists). Of these, nearly half practise acupuncture (mainly doctors and physiotherapists), about a quarter practise reflexology (mainly nurses and midwives), and about one in seven practise homeopathy (mainly doctors, chiropodists, and podiatrists). Many more conventional healthcare professionals, especially general practitioners, have attended basic training courses and provide limited forms of complementary medicine without official registration.

Complementary medicine provided by the NHS

A substantial amount of complementary medicine is provided by conventional healthcare professionals within existing NHS services. An estimated 4.2 million adults made 22 million visits to practitioners of one of the six established therapies in 1998, with 90% of this purchased privately. However, the NHS provided an estimated 10% of these contacts (2 million). A UK-wide survey in 1995 showed that almost 40% of all general practices offered some form of access to complementary medicine for their NHS patients, of which over 70% was paid for by the NHS. This survey was repeated in 2001 and showed that one in two practices in England now offer their patients some access to complementary medicine; however, the range of complementary services on offer is narrow, perhaps only a single type of treatment being offered. Over half of these practices provided complementary medicine via a member of the primary healthcare team, usually a general practitioner.

Less is known about access via secondary care, but certain specialties are more likely to provide complementary therapies. In 1998, a survey of hospices revealed that over 90% offered some complementary therapy to patients. Pain clinics, oncology units, and rehabilitation wards also often provide complementary therapies.

Further reading

Coward R. *The Whole Truth*. London: Faber and Faber, 1989.

Fisher P, Ward A. Complementary medicine in Europe. *BMJ* 1994; **309**: 107–11.

Furnham A. Why do people choose and use complementary therapies? In: Ernst E, ed. *Complementary Medicine, an objective appraisal*. Oxford: Butterworth Heinemann, 1998; 71–88.

Mills S, Budd S. *Professional Organisation of Complementary and Alternative Medicine in the United Kingdom. A second report to the Department of Health*. Exeter: University of Exeter, 2000.

Mills S, Peacock W. *Professional Organisation of Complementary and Alternative Medicine in the United Kingdom 1997: a report to the Department of Health*. Exeter: Centre for Complementary Health Studies, University of Exeter, 1997.

Partnership on Long-term Conditions. *17 Million Reasons: improving the lives of people with longterm conditions*. Partnership on Long-term Conditions, 2005, www.17millionreasons.org.

Sharma U. *Complementary Medicine Today: practitioners and patients*, revised edn. London: Routledge, 1995.

Thomas KJ, Coleman P. Use of complementary or alternative medicine in a general population in Great Britain. *J Pub Health* 2004; **25**(2): 152–5.

Thomas KJ, Coleman P, Nicholl JP. Trends in access to complementary and alternative medicines via primary care in England: 1995–2001. Results from a follow-up national survey. *Fam Pract* 2003; **20**: 575–7.

Thomas KJ, Fall M, Parry G, Nicholl J. *National Survey of Access to Complementary Health Care via General Practice: report to Department of Health*. Sheffield: SCHARR, 1995.

Thomas KJ, Nicholl JP, Coleman P. Use and expenditure on complementary medicine in England: a population based survey. *Complement Ther Med* 2001; **9**: 2–11.

Wearn AM, Greenfield SM. Access to complementary medicine in general practice: survey in one UK health authority. *J Roy Soc Med* 1998; **91**: 465–70.

CHAPTER 3

Complementary/Integrated Medicine in Conventional Practice

Catherine Zollman, Jane Wilkinson, Amanda Nadin, and Eleanor Lines

The past 15 years has seen a significant increase in the amount of complementary and alternative medicine (CAM) being accessed through the NHS. These services are not evenly distributed, and many different delivery mechanisms are used, some of which (such as homeopathic hospitals) predate the inception of the NHS. Others depend on more recent NHS reorganizations, like general practice-based and Primary Care Trust (PCT) commissioning, or have been set up as evaluated pilot projects.

In general, the development of these services has been demand led rather than evidence led. A few have published formal evaluations or audit reports. Some of these show benefits associated with complementary therapy – high patient satisfaction, significant improvements on validated health questionnaires compared with waiting list controls, and suggestions of reduced prescribing and referrals. These pilot projects have also identified various factors that influence the integration of complementary medicine practitioners within NHS settings. However, evidence suggests that positive service evaluations in CAM do not necessarily secure future funding from commissioners.

Perspectives on integration

The term 'integrated health care' is often used to describe the provision of complementary therapies within an NHS setting. However, this provision often takes different forms, so, for example, a massage therapist may be integral to a multidisciplinary team within a palliative care setting. In contrast, a GP may refer patients to an osteopath within a PCT, but have very little contact with the practitioner.

Conventional clinicians and managers want persuasive evidence that complementary medicine can deliver safe, cost-effective solutions to problems that are expensive or difficult to manage with conventional treatment. A moderate number of randomized trials and a few reliable economic analyses of complementary medicine have been conducted. Systematic processes for collecting data on safety and adverse events are only in their infancy.

While much-needed evidence is gathered, the debate about more widespread integration of complementary medicine continues. The idea of providing such care within a framework of evidence-based medicine, NHS reorganizations, and healthcare rationing raises various concerns for the different parties involved.

Box 3.1 Examples of cost–benefit analyses of integrated CAM projects

Glastonbury Health Centre, Somerset
Glastonbury Health Centre is a rural, integrated general practice working towards practice-based commissioning. Over 600 patients were referred to the service during the 3-year evaluation period (1994–1997) – approximately 17% of the practice population. The evaluation was conducted in-house using validated outcome tools including the SF-36 20 and the Functional Limitation Profile and Pain Index (Hills & Welford 1998).
- Outcomes reported 6 months after CAM treatment:
  - 85% patients referred reported an improvement in their condition following treatment
  - 85% also reported being satisfied with the treatment they received
- Cost savings:
  - there was a reduction in referrals to secondary care
  - there was a reduction in usage of other health services (GP time, prescriptions, X-rays, and other tests)

Newcastle Primary Care Trust
Newcastle Primary Care Trust is an integrated health service across a New Deal for Communities locality. More than 650 patients were seen over the 3-year evaluation period (2001–2004). Evaluation was undertaken independently by the University of Northumbria (Carmichael 2004).
- Patient satisfaction:
  - 96% patients were satisfied with the service
  - 62% were extremely satisfied with the service
  - patient satisfaction surveys showed that 83% of patients reported they did not need any further treatment from their GP during the treatment period and for 6 months afterwards
- Estimated cost savings:
  - there was a 39% reduction in prescriptions 6 months after CAM treatment, representing a cost saving of £4800
  - there was a 31% reduction in the number of GP consultations, representing a cost difference of £10 000
  - the total estimated savings make up 40% of the total project costs

Modified from Thomson (2005).

Patients

Public surveys show that most people support increased provision of complementary medicine on the NHS, but this question is often asked in isolation and does not mean that patients would necessarily prefer complementary to conventional care. Patients also want to be protected from unqualified complementary practitioners and inappropriate treatments. NHS provision might go some way to ensuring certain minimum standards such as proper regulation, standardized note keeping, effective channels of communication, and participation in research. It would also facilitate ongoing medical assessment. By applying the same clinical governance as for conventional practices within the NHS, complementary medicine can begin to gain acceptability.

Complementary practitioners

Some practitioners support NHS provision because it would improve equity of access, protect their right to practise (currently vulnerable to changes in European and national legislation), and guarantee a caseload. It would also provide opportunities for inter-professional learning, career development, and research. Some are concerned about the possibility of loss of autonomy, poorer working conditions, and domination by the medical model.

Current provision in the NHS

In primary care

Most of the complementary medicine provided through the NHS is delivered in primary care.

Direct provision

Over 20% of primary healthcare teams provide some form of complementary therapy directly. For example, general practitioners may use homeopathy, and practice nurses may use hypnosis or reflexology. The advantages of this system are that it requires minimal financial investment and that complementary treatments are usually offered only after conventional assessment and diagnosis. Also, practitioners can monitor patients from a conventional viewpoint, ensure compliance with essential conventional medication, and identify interactions and adverse events.

A disadvantage is that shorter appointments may leave less time for non-specific aspects of the therapeutic consultation. Also,

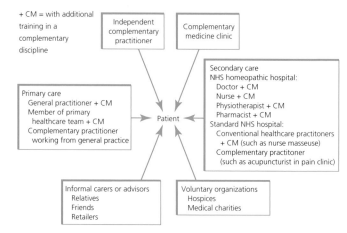

Figure 3.1 Model of the provision of complementary medicine.

members of primary healthcare teams have often undertaken only a basic training in complementary medicine, and this generally forms only a small part of their work. Doubts about the effectiveness of the complementary treatments they deliver, compared with those given by full-time complementary therapists, have been expressed. Although no comparative evidence is available, it is clear that limits of competence need to be recognized.

As levels of professionalism improve within the CAM field, GPs may be more prepared to delegate patients to CAM practitioners but this will obviously have funding implications.

Indirect provision

Complementary practitioners without a background in conventional health care work in at least 20% of UK general practices. Osteopathy is the most commonly encountered profession. Such practitioners usually work privately, but some are employed by the practice and function as ancillary staff. An advantage for patients is that the general practice usually checks practitioners' references and credentials. Although some guidelines for referral may exist, levels of communication with GPs vary widely and levels of integration vary with the practice.

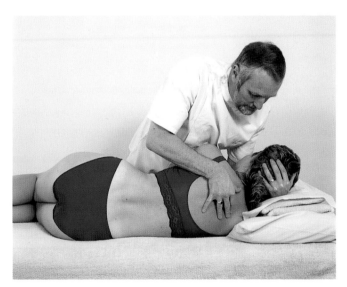

Figure 3.2 In many general practices, osteopathy is provided indirectly by an independent complementary practitioner. Reproduced with permission of the General Osteopathic Council.

In specialist provider units

Five NHS homeopathic hospitals across the UK accept referrals from primary care under normal NHS conditions: free at the point of care. They offer a variety of complementary therapies provided by conventionally trained health professionals. They provide opportunities for large-scale audit and evaluation of complementary medicine, but many services have been cut in recent years and those that still exist are under constant threat in the current climate of evidence-based healthcare rationing.

Some independent complementary medicine centres have contracts with local NHS purchasers. For example, in the late 1990s Wessex Health Authority contracted a private clinic to provide a multidisciplinary package of complementary medicine for NHS patients with chronic fatigue or hyperactivity. Some PCTs have commissioned CAM from independent centres such as local chiropractic clinics rather than employ complementary practitioners directly. A few health authorities have set up pilot projects for multidisciplinary complementary medicine clinics in the community or on hospital premises. Advantages have included clear referral guidelines, evaluation, good communication with GPs, and supervised and accountable complementary practitioners. However, such centres are particularly vulnerable when health authorities come under financial pressure. Examples are the Liverpool Centre for Health and the former Lewisham Hospital NHS Trust Complementary Therapy Centre, which was closed when the local health authority had to reduce its overspend.

In conventional secondary care

Many NHS hospital trusts offer some form of complementary medicine to patients. This may be provided by practitioners with or without backgrounds in conventional health care (Table 3.1). However, the availability of such services varies widely and depends heavily on local interest and high level support.

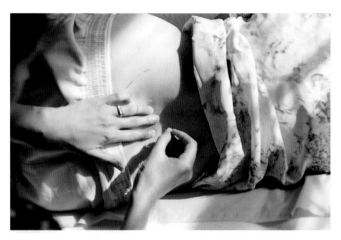

Figure 3.3 An increasing number of hospital pain clinics now offer acupuncture as a treatment for chronic pain. Reproduced with permission of the Royal London Homeopathic Hospital.

Commissioning complementary therapies within the NHS

Recent financial reforms within the NHS are being driven by policies that are designed to devolve decision-making power from Whitehall, increase the plurality of service providers, and improve patients' ability to choose where, when and how they are treated. These policies also shift the focus of health care towards the treatment of long-term conditions. The changes in contracting and financial flows are intended to support the implementation of these policies and may, in the future, make it easier to commission complementary therapies (Table 3.2).

Table 3.1 Examples of complementary medicine in secondary care.

Complementary therapy	Healthcare professionals
● **Pain clinics**	
Acupuncture	Anaesthetists, physiotherapists, palliative care physicians, professional acupuncturists
● **Physiotherapy departments**	
Manipulative therapy, acupuncture	Physiotherapists trained in manipulative medicine or acupuncture
● **Rheumatology departments**	
Manipulative therapy	Osteopaths, chiropractors, orthopaedic physicians
● **Hospices**	
Aromatherapy, reflexology, massage, hypnosis, relaxation, healing, acupuncture, homeopathy	Nurses, doctors, complementary therapists, occupational therapists
● **Clinical psychology departments**	
Hypnosis or relaxation training	Psychologists
● **Obstetric departments**	
Yoga, acupuncture	Midwives, physiotherapists
● **Drug and alcohol services**	
Acupuncture (ofter auricular)	Mental health workers, drug workers, professional acupuncturists

Table 3.2 NHS primary care contracts (England).

Contract	Implications for complementary health care
Practice-based commissioning (PBC)	Practices will have greater autonomy in terms of deciding what sort of services they offer for their patients Holding a budget will allow them to offer patients a choice of complementary treatments, which may be attractive as a cheaper alternative
Payment by results (PbR)	Money released by more rational use of referrals, diagnostics, and prescribing may be put in to complementary health services
New general medical services (nGMS)	GP partners can employ a range of healthcare professionals Enhanced services provide some funding for specialist/local provision
Personal medical services (PMS)	Flexible services and workforce Alternative quality and outcomes framework (QOF) available
Specialist personal medical services (SPMS)	Flexible services and workforce PCTs could commission CAMs directly using SPMS
Alternative provider medical services (APMS)	Specialist service possible Will increase the range of healthcare practitioners/providers who can deliver services as many complementary practitioners operate in the private sector
Primary care trust medical services (PCTMS)	Directly commissioned by PCT Specialist service possible Allows individuals to approach PCT

Modified from Thomson (2005).

Within the new financial system patients could, in theory, choose complementary therapy options over conventional care and money should follow those patients. The reforms are a huge overhaul of NHS current financial systems and are going to place obvious challenges on those that implement them, but they also represent a great opportunity for those working at the frontline of health care in facilitating innovative service redesign.

Primary care contracting

In theory, PCTs can commission CAM services through general medical services (GMS) and personal medical services (PMS) contracts via the locally enhanced services mechanism, but currently the lack of available resources within the system often makes it difficult to fund new developments as well as provide essential services. Another way that CAM therapies can be provided to a local population is via the PCT medical services (PCTMS) contract, which enables PCTs to directly commission non-NHS service providers. The launch of alternative provider medical services (APMS) contracts and practice-based commissioning (PBC) represent the most interesting developments for GPs wishing to integrate CAMs.

Alternative provider medical services

Introduced in 2004, APMS contracts allow PCTs to commission from a wide range of providers. PCTs can contract with any individual or organization that meets the service provider conditions and clinical governance requirements; this includes the independent and voluntary sectors, not-for-profit organizations, and NHS organizations. The contract has been specifically designed to be flexible and responsive to local needs, giving PCTs the freedom to develop new ways of improving capacity and shaping services. The use of APMS for commissioning CAM could provide PCTs and GPs with different options for managing long term conditions, improving patient choice and responsiveness, as well as tackling capacity issues and effectiveness gaps. For a variety of reasons, uptake of the APMS contract within primary care has been slow and some GPs are concerned that APMS will lead to the privatization of the NHS.

Practice-based commissioning

The implementation of PBC is perhaps the most likely means for integrating CAM within primary care. Since April 2005, every GP practice has been able to hold a PBC budget. Signing up has been voluntary and in December 2006 the Department of Health reported that universal coverage of PBC had been achieved. Unlike previous contracting systems, savings made through effective commissioning can be reinvested for developing patient services, including complementary medicine. Practices can also choose to work in networks to improve efficiency and to work together in areas of service redesign. The PCTs' role will be to manage contracts, procurement processes, and provide back office functions such as payment processing.

It is difficult to gauge how APMS contracts and PBC will affect the uptake of CAM services, as they are still fairly new and untested for the CAM field, but under the current contracting system the provision of CAM within the NHS is increasing. A recent study indicates that patients in 59% of PCTs have access to CAM via primary care (Wilkinson *et al.* 2004). It remains to be seen whether complementary medicine will be identified as a priority by sufficiently large numbers of primary care-based and PCT commissioners to enable the creation of any new initiatives.

Other ways of funding complementary medicine in NHS primary care

Complementary medicine can also be provided by conventional NHS healthcare professionals as part of everyday clinical care. This requires no special funding arrangements but obviously needs to be balanced with other uses of their time. For example, general practitioners may provide basic acupuncture or homeopathy within standard appointments. Nurses and midwives may use relaxation techniques or simple massage in settings as diverse as intensive care and maternity units.

Local and national government regeneration monies (e.g. New Deal for Communities) have sometimes been used to finance free complementary medicine in deprived areas such as inner city Nottingham (the Impact Integrated Medicine Partnership) and Bristol (formerly CHIPS, now the Bristol Complementary Health Clinic). However, once the time-limited regeneration money runs out, these services usually have to start charging for treatments.

Funds from the voluntary sector or charities may also be sought. The complementary therapy service at the Marylebone Health Centre in London was initially funded by a research grant from a charitable trust. Fundraising and donations by the local patients

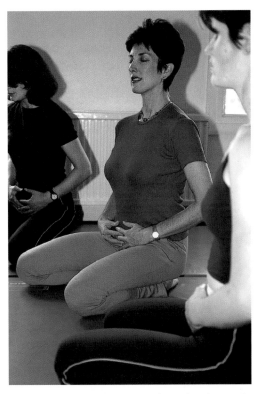

Figure 3.4 Some complementary therapies, such as relaxation, can be delivered effectively in group sessions, which may contribute to cost savings. Reproduced with permission of BMJ/Ulrike Preuss.

are now essential to its ongoing financial viability. Some charities provide free CAM treament for defined patient groups and liaise with local health services. Unfortunately such funding is precarious and these initiatives are often short lived or very small-scale operations. Hospices, which normally receive charitable funding support, are now almost all able to offer some form of complementary therapy.

Many occupational health and private medical insurance schemes fund a limited range of complementary therapies.

Governance and standards in complementary and alternative medicine

Complementary practitioners are working within their professional associations to improve standards of training and practice, with the aim of assuring accountability to both patients and NHS commissioners about the quality and safety of their services.

The processes of clinical governance (CG) are as applicable to CAM practice as they are to conventional medicine. Future NHS access to CAM will depend on ensuring adequate structures for evaluating, monitoring, and assuring standards of care. The value of clinical governance is that it provides a universal framework for professional development, quality improvement, and accountability.

Evidence-based practice

As has occurred within primary care, developing an evidence base for under-researched interventions has been a focus for improving

Box 3.4 **Key evaluation reports from NHS complementary medicine services**

Canter PH, Coon JT, Ernst E. Cost-effectiveness of complementary therapies in the United Kingdom – a systematic review. *Evidence Based Complement Altern Med* 2006; **3**(4): 425–32.

Hills D, Welford R. *Complementary Therapy in General Practice: an evaluation of the Glastonbury Health Centre Complementary Medicine Service.* Glastonbury, Somerset: Somerset Trust for Integrated Health Care, 1998.

Hotchkiss J. *Liverpool Centre for Health: the first year of a service offering complementary therapies on the NHS.* Observatory Report Series No. 25. Liverpool: Liverpool Public Health Observatory, 1995.

Rees R. Evaluating complementary therapy on the NHS: a critique of reports from three pilot projects. *Complement Ther Med* 1996; **4**: 254–7.

Robertson, F. *Impact Integrated Medicine Project: annual report.* Nottingham: Waverley Health Centre, 2005, www.impact-imp. co.uk.

Scheurmier N, Breen AC. A pilot study of the purchase of manipulation services for acute low back pain in the United Kingdom. *Manipulative Physiol Ther* 1998; **21**: 14–18.

Spence DS, Thompson EA, Barron SJ. Homeopathic treatment for chronic disease: a 6-year, university-hospital outpatient observational study. *J Altern Complement Med* 2005; **11**(5): 793–8.

Wye L, Shaw A, Sharp D. Evaluating complementary and alternative therapy services in primary and community care settings: a review of 25 services. *Complement Ther Med* 2006; **14**: 220–30.

Box 3.5 **Web resources**

- iCAM online – a knowledge business development network for the complementary and integrated healthcare sectors, providing access to an online community, courses and events as well as resources on clinical governance, service and business development
  URL: http://www.icamonline.org.uk
- National Library for Health Specialist Library for Complementary and Alternative Medicine – launched in May 2006
  URL: http://www.library.nhs.uk/cam
- Complementary and Alternative Medicine Evidence On-Line (CAMEOL) – coordinated by the Research Council for Complementary Medicine (RCCM), University of Westminster, and University of Plymouth. Provides a review and critical appraisal of published research in specific complementary therapies, focusing on key areas of NHS priority
  URL: http://www.rccm.org.uk/cameol
- National Centre for Complementary and Alternative Medicine (NCCAM) – part of the National Institutes of Health (USA), providing research resources and reviews
  URL: http://www.nccam.nih.gov
- Royal London Homeopathic Hospital (RLHH) CAM Information Centre – walk-in centre providing information on complementary and alternative medicine for the public and healthcare practitioners
  URL: http://www.uclh.nhs.uk
- Natural Medicines Database – comprehensive details of herbs, contraindications and pharmacovigilence
  URL: http://www.naturaldatabase.com
- Medicines and Healthcare products Regulatory Agency (MHRA)
  URL: http://www.mhra.gov.uk
- NHS Primary Care contracting – works across the NHS and other relevant organisations to support primary care commissioners in the develpoment of primary care. They provide support and guidance, which aims to maximize the benefits of the new contracts in primary medical care, pharmacy, dentistry, practice based commissioning, optometry and innovation/extending services in primary care
  URL: http://www.primarycarecontracting.nhs.uk
- Research Council for Complementary Medicine (RCCM)
  URL: http://www.rccm.org.uk

quality and establishing standards. The evidence base for CAM is beginning to develop as research capacity increases. New initiatives for reviewing and accessing data will enable evaluations of cost effectiveness, practical research, and audit activity, including benchmarking and standard setting. Recent research has begun to demonstrate cost savings through reductions in prescribing rates and demands on conventional practitioner time.

Intelligent use of information

Information systems are essential for providing assurances on safety and quality as well as providing feedback to shape services within the NHS. If they are to integrate within the NHS, complementary practitioners will need to adhere to policies and guidelines relating to confidentiality, use of information, and informed consent and have an understanding of NHS technology systems. Equally, PCTs need information on complementary medicine so that commissioners can select and locate services of high quality.

Patient focus

CAM practitioners aim to provide patient-centred holistic and individual packages of care. Aspects of self-care such as exercise, relaxation techniques, and nutritional advice are present in many complementary approaches and may have the potential to address the government's agendas on public health, choice, and chronic disease management.

Patient safety

Ensuring patient safety is central to clinical governance. Local and national initiatives have begun to introduce systems for collating and monitoring incidents, trigger events and trends in relation to complementary therapies. Protocols are being developed for the prevention and control of specific risks, for example counting in and out the needles in acupuncture, or the safe storage of aromatherapy oils. The Medicines Healthcare Regulatory Authority has an advisory group on herbal medicines and homeopathy and a yellow card scheme exists for reporting adverse reactions and for pharmacovigilance. Further work will be necessary for developing coherent risk policies and procedures for CAM, as well as comprehensive strategies for implementation.

Education and staffing

Educational standards are being raised with the expansion of university courses and through the introduction of National

Occupational Standards for CAM. Continuing professional development is incorporated within the regulatory frameworks for statutory and voluntary self-regulatory bodies. Governance will be facilitated by involving practitioners in mainstream educational programmes, holding multidisciplinary meetings, and by practitioners incorporating aspects of service development plans within their own personal development plans. The Royal College of General Practitioner's Quality Team Development Scheme initiative can be adapted for complementary approaches to facilitate participation in clinical governance and the provision of more integrated services.

Future governance of complementary therapies

The type and range of CG activities required for NHS provision of CAM will depend on the type of healthcare setting (e.g. primary care, community, hospital). Established services such as the Royal London Homeopathic Hospital have well-developed CG systems and processes that are aligned to its parent organization, the University College Hospital London NHS Foundation Trust. The statutorily regulated professions of chiropractic and osteopathy have already established quality improvement programmes and other highly organized CAM professions, such as acupuncture, herbal medicine and homeopathy, have made significant advances. As the regulation of other CAM disciplines progresses, CG will be incorporated into registration requirements and continuing professional development. Additionally, integrated governance frameworks will need to be applied to CAM practice, and CAM practitioners will need to consider working to standards monitored by the Healthcare Commission. Work in this area has been supported by Department of Health investment in clinical governance for CAM, regulation and research infrastructure.

Further reading

British Medical Association. *General Practitioners Committee Guidance for GPs: referrals to complementary therapists.* London: BMA, 1999, http://www.osteopathy.org.uk/integrated_health/bma_referral.pdf.

Carmichael S. *PCT Complementary Therapy Project Evaluation Report for New Deal for Communities.* 2004.

Coates J, Jobst K. Integrated healthcare, a way forward for the next five years? *Altern Complement Med* 1998; **4**: 209–47.

Fulder S. *The Handbook of Alternative and Complementary Medicine,* 3rd edn. Oxford: Oxford University Press, 1996.

Hills D, Welford R. *Complementary Therapy in General Practice: an evaluation of the Glastonbury Health Centre complementary medicine service, 1998.* http://www.integratedhealth.org.uk/report.html.

Peters D, Chaitow L, Harris G, Morrison S. *Integrating Complementary Therapies in Primary Care: a practical guide for health professionals.* Edinburgh: Churchill Livingstone, 2001.

Pinder MZ. *Complementary Healthcare: a guide for patients.* London: The Prince of Wales's Foundation for Integrated Health, 2005.

Sharma U. *Complementary Medicine Today: practitioners and patients,* revised edn. London: Routledge, 1995.

Stone J, Matthews J. *Complementary Medicine and the Law.* Oxford: Oxford University Press, 1996.

Tavares M. *National Guidelines for the use of Complementary Therapies in Supportive and Palliative Care.* London: The Prince of Wales's Foundation for Integrated Health, May 2003.

Thomson A. *A Healthy Partnership: integrating complementary healthcare into primary care.* London: The Prince of Wales's Foundation for Integrated Health, 2005.

Wilkinson J, Peters D, Donaldson J, Nadin A. *Clinical Governance for CAM in Primary Care: final report to the Department of Health and King's Fund, October 2004.* London: University of Westminster, 2004.

CHAPTER 4

Acupuncture

Catherine Zollman and Andrew Vickers

Acupuncture is the stimulation of special points on the body, usually by the insertion of fine needles. Originating in the Far East about 2000 years ago, it has made various appearances in the history of European and North American medicine. William Osler, for example, used acupuncture therapeutically in the 19th century. Acupuncture's recent popularity in the West dates from the 1970s, when President Nixon visited China.

Background

In its original form acupuncture was based on the principles of traditional Chinese medicine. According to these, the workings of the human body are controlled by a vital force or energy called 'Qi' (pronounced 'chee'), which circulates between the organs along channels called meridians.

There are 12 main meridians, and these correspond to 12 major functions or 'organs' of the body. Although they have the same names (such as liver, kidney, heart, etc.), Chinese and Western concepts of the organs correlate only very loosely. Qi energy must flow in the correct strength and quality through each of these meridians and organs for health to be maintained. The acupuncture points are located along the meridians and provide one means of altering the flow of Qi.

Although the details of practice may differ between individual schools, all traditional acupuncture theory is based in the Daoist concept of yin and yang. Illness is seen in terms of excesses or deficiencies in various exogenous and endogenous pathogenic factors, and treatment is aimed at restoring balance. Traditional diagnoses are esoteric, such as 'kidney-yang deficiency, water overflowing' or 'damp heat in the bladder'.

Many of the conventional health professionals who practise acupuncture have dispensed with such concepts. Acupuncture points are seen to correspond to physiological and anatomical features such as peripheral nerve junctions, and diagnosis is made in purely conventional terms. An important concept used by such acupuncturists is that of the 'trigger point' (called 'Ah Shee' in traditional acupuncture). This is an area of increased sensitivity within a muscle, which is said to cause a characteristic pattern of referred pain in a related segment of the body. An example might be tender areas in the muscles of the neck and shoulder that relate to various patterns of headache.

It is often implied that a clear and firm distinction exists between traditional and Western acupuncture, but the two approaches overlap considerably. Moreover, traditional acupuncture is not a single, historically stable therapy. There are many different schools – for example, Japanese practitioners differ from their Chinese counterparts by using mainly shallow needle insertion.

Acupressure involves firm manual pressure on selected acupuncture points. Shiatsu, a modified form of acupressure, was systematized as part of traditional Japanese medicine.

How does acupuncture work?

The effects of acupuncture, particularly on pain, are at least partially explicable within a conventional physiological model. Acupuncture is known to stimulate $A\delta$ fibres entering the dorsal horn of the spinal cord. These mediate segmental inhibition of pain impulses carried in the slower, unmyelinated C fibres and, through connections in the midbrain, enhance descending inhibition of C fibre pain impulses at other levels of the spinal cord. This helps explain why acupuncture needles in one part of the body can affect pain sensation in another region. Acupuncture is also known to stimulate release of endogenous opioids and other neurotransmitters such as serotonin. This is likely to be another mechanism for acupuncture's effects, such as in acute pain and in substance misuse.

However, certain aspects of traditional acupuncture, which have some empirical support, resist conventional explanation. In one unreplicated study, for example, blinded assessment of the tenderness of points on the ear had high agreement with the true location of chronic pain in distant parts of the body. Changes in the electrical conductivity of acupuncture points associated with a particular organ have also been recorded in patients with corresponding conventional diseases. Acupuncture points have been demonstrated to have reproducibly different skin impedance from surrounding skin areas. There are no sufficient anatomical or physiological explanations for these observations.

What happens during a treatment?

Traditional acupuncturists supplement a detailed, multisystem case history with observations that are said to give information

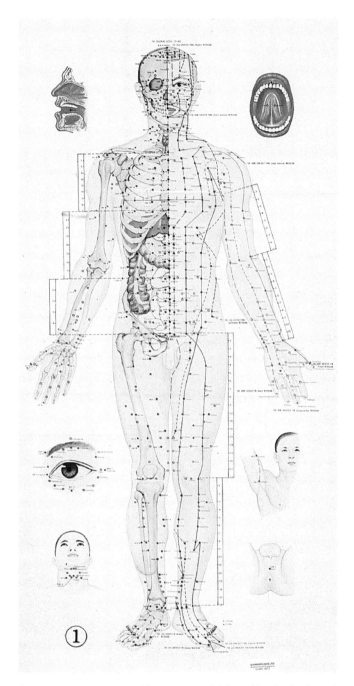

Figure 4.1 Accupuncture meridians run superficially and longitudinally. Both traditional and Western acupuncturists identify acupuncture points by their location on the meridian – for example, gall bladder 30 or large intestine 4. Reproduced with permission of Medicine and Health Publishing, Hong Kong, and supplied by Scarboroughs.

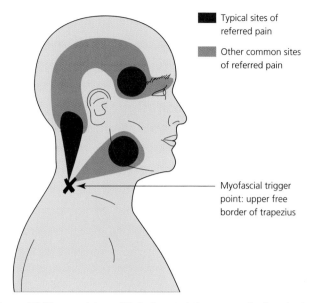

Figure 4.2 Trigger points, and their characteristic patterns of referred pain, can be treated by direct needling at the trigger point. This concept is also used in musculoskeletal medicine, with trigger points being treated by manipulative techniques. Supplied by Mike Cummings of the British Medical Acupuncture Society.

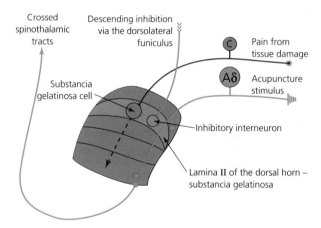

Figure 4.3 The neuronal connections that are thought to mediate the effects of acupuncture on pain. Supplied by Mike Cummings of the British Medical Acupuncture Society.

about the patient's state of health. These include examination of the shape, coating, and colour of the tongue; the colour of the face; and the strength, rhythm, and quality of the pulse. Both Western and traditional practitioners may palpate to identify points at which pressure causes tenderness or pain.

Typically, between four and 10 points are needled during an acupuncture session. The needles are usually left in place for 10–30 minutes, although some practitioners needle for only a few seconds or minutes. Needles may be stimulated by manual twirling or a small electric current. Lasers are sometimes used to stimulate acupuncture points instead of needles. Acupuncture needles are extremely fine and do not hurt in the same way as, say, an injection. Patients may even be unaware that a needle has been inserted. However, some acupuncturists attempt to produce a sensation called 'de Qi' – a sense of heaviness, warmth, soreness, or numbness at the point of needling. This is said to be a sign that an acupuncture point has been correctly stimulated. Many patients say that they find acupuncture a relaxing or sedating experience.

Traditional acupuncturists may use various adjunctive therapies, including moxibustion (the burning of a herb just above the surface of the skin), massage, cupping, herbal preparations, exercises, and dietary modification.

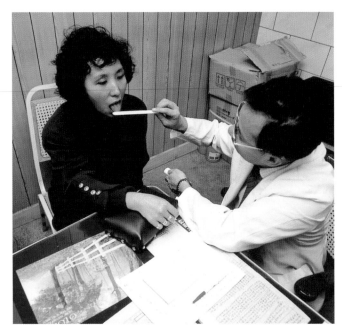

Figure 4.4 A typical traditional acupuncture session includes a physical assessment of yin yang energy status with methods such as pulse and tongue diagnosis. Reproduced with permission of Mark de Fraye/Science Photo Library.

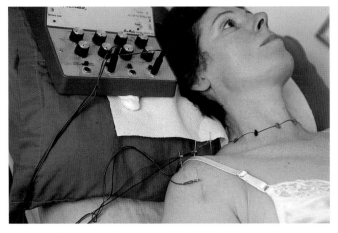

Figure 4.5 Using electricity to stimulate acupuncture points is thought to augment the therapeutic effect of needling and is used particularly in treating chronic pain. Reproduced with permission of BMJ/Ulrike Press.

A typical course of acupuncture treatment for a chronic condition would be six to 12 sessions over a 3-month period. This might be followed by 'top up' treatments every 2–6 months.

Increasingly, self-acupuncture is being introduced using semipermanent needles, studs, or self-needling of specific limited points.

Therapeutic scope

Acupuncture was developed as a relatively global system of medicine. Some current textbooks refer to treating conditions as varied as diarrhoea, the common cold, and tinnitus. As practised in Europe and North America, acupuncture is primarily a treatment for benign, chronic disease and for musculoskeletal injury. The most common presenting complaints found in surveys of acupuncture practice include back pain, arthritis, headache, asthma, hay fever, anxiety, fatigue, menstrual disorders, and digestive disorders. Acupuncture is also used in drug and alcohol rehabilitation, particularly in the United States.

Research evidence

There is good research evidence that acupuncture has effects greater than placebo. Randomized trials have generally, though not always, found that true acupuncture is more effective in relieving pain than a 'sham' technique, such as inserting needles away from true points. Of the numerous studies on nausea, a condition that readily lends itself to placebo controlled trials, almost all show that stimulating true acupuncture points is more effective that stimulating false points.

> Box 4.1 **Key studies of efficacy**
>
> Furlan AD, van Tulder MW, Cherkin DC, Tsukayama H, Lao L, Koes BW, Berman BM. Acupuncture and dry-needling for low back pain. *Cochrane Database Syst Rev* 2005; **1**: CD001351.
>
> Lee A, Done ML. Stimulation of the wrist acupuncture point P6 for preventing postoperative nausea and vomiting. *Cochrane Database Syst Rev* 2004; **3**: CD003281.
>
> Vickers AJ, Rees RW, Zollman CE, *et al*. Acupuncture for chronic headache in primary care: large, pragmatic, randomised trial. *BMJ* 2004; **328**(7442): 744.
>
> White AR, Rampes H, Campbell JL. Acupuncture and related interventions for smoking cessation. *Cochrane Database Syst Rev* 2006; **1**: CD000009.

Acupuncture has clinically important benefits for pain conditions such as migraine, osteoarthritis, and low back pain. Several large, 'pragmatic' trials have found that patients receiving acupuncture have lower pain scores at long-term follow-up than patients receiving usual medical care alone.

The evidence is far less clear for conditions treated by acupuncturists in routine practice other than pain. There are conflicting results from a small number of trials for asthma, hay fever, substance abuse, mood disorder, and menopausal symptoms. Systematic reviews and randomized controlled trials suggest that acupuncture is probably not of benefit for stopping smoking, tinnitus, or obesity.

There is little reliable information on the relative effectiveness of the various Western and traditional forms of acupuncture.

Safety

Acupuncture is a relatively safe form of treatment with a very low incidence of serious adverse events. Several prospective studies examining acupuncture safety have included very large numbers

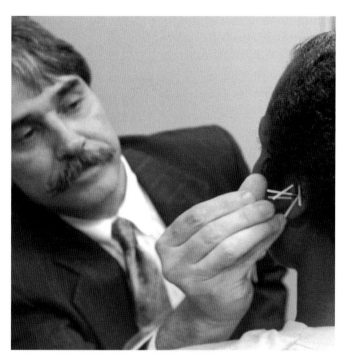

Figure 4.6 On balance, research evidence supports the use of acupuncture in treating substance misuse. Auricular acupuncture is often used for this purpose. Reproduced with permission of AP/Shane Young.

of treatments (e.g. 55 000 or 34 000 treatments) and no serious adverse events have been reported. An extensive worldwide literature search identified only 193 adverse events (including relatively minor events such as bruising and dizziness) over 15 years. The more serious events were usually related to poor practice – for example, cases of hepatitis B infection typically involved bad hygiene and unregistered practitioners. Nonetheless, there have been case reports of serious adverse events such as pneumothorax or spinal lesions.

Box 4.2 **Key studies of safety**

MacPherson H., Thomas K. Short term reactions to acupuncture – a cross-sectional survey of patient reports. *Acupuncture Med* 2005; **23**(3): 112–20.

White A. A cumulative review of the range and incidence of significant adverse events associated with acupuncture. *Acupuncture Med* 2004; **22**(3): 122–33.

Indwelling 'press' needles are commonly used in the treatment of addiction and should be used with care. They have been associated with infections such as perichondritis. Systemic infection seems to be very uncommon, but acupuncture should probably be avoided in patients with valvular heart defects.

Practitioners

Acupuncturists without a background in conventional health care tend to work in private practice and treat a wide variety of conditions. About 2000 doctors and physiotherapists in the UK practise acupuncture, but they rarely specialize in it and generally use it as an adjunctive treatment when appropriate. Most offer treatment mainly directed at musculoskeletal and other painful conditions and are usually based in pain clinics or in general practice.

Training

Professional acupuncturists train for up to 3–4 years full time and may acquire university degrees on completion of their training. Some complete further training in the principles and practice of Chinese herbalism. All accredited acupuncture training courses include conventional anatomy, physiology, pathology, and diagnosis. Research and audit skills are also taught.

Medical acupuncturists generally have fewer training hours in acupuncture techniques – a course of several weekends in which they learn a small range of simple techniques is typical. Other conventional healthcare disciplines run courses for their own members, ranging from basic introductions to 2-year training in advanced acupuncture.

Regulation

Professional acupuncturists have a single regulatory body, the British Acupuncture Council (BAcC), with more than 2500 members. All members have undergone a training independently accredited by the British Acupuncture Accreditation Board. The government has established a joint acupuncture and herbal medicine working group to progress joint statutory regulation of these professions. Physiotherapists are regulated by the Acupuncture Association of Chartered Physiotherapists (AACP). Although many doctors practise some basic acupuncture without an official qualification, most have done at least a short course approved by the British Medical Acupuncture Society. This society also offers a Certificate of Basic Competence and a Diploma of Medical Acupuncture for appropriately trained doctors. In the near future a masters level qualification will also be offered.

Box 4. 3 **Training and regulatory organizations**

- British Medical Acupuncture Society (BMAS): for doctors only
  BMAS House, 3 Winnington Court, Northwich, Cheshire CW8 1AQ, UK. Tel: 0160 678 6782; fax: 01606 786783; email: Admin@ medical-acupuncture.org.uk; URL: http://www.medical-acupuncture.co.uk
- British Acupuncture Council
  63 Jeddo Road, London W12 9HQ, UK. Tel: 0208 735 0400; fax: 020 8735 0404; URL: http://www.acupuncture.org.uk
- Acupuncture Association of Chartered Physiotherapists AACP Limited
  Southgate House, Southgate Park, Bakewell Road, Orton Southgate, Peterborough PE2 6YS, UK. Tel 0173 339 0012; URL: http://www.aacp.uk.com

---

Further reading

Acupuncture Resource Research Centre Website, www.acupunctureresearch.org.uk

Campbell A. *Acupuncture in Practice*, 2nd edn. Oxford: Butterworth Heinemann, 2004.

Filshie J, White A. *Medical Acupuncture*. Edinburgh: Churchill Livingstone, 1997.

Hopwood V. *Acupuncture in Physiotherapy: Key Concepts and Evidence-Based Practice*. Oxford: Butterworth Heinemann, 2004.

Kaptchuk T. *Chinese Medicine: The Web that has no Weaver*. London: Rider, 1983.

Maciocia G. *The Foundations of Chinese Medicine*. Edinburgh: Churchill Livingstone, 1989.

MacPherson H, Kaptchuk TJ, eds. *Acupuncture in Practice Case History Insights from the West*. Edinburgh: Churchill Livingstone, 1996.

CHAPTER 5

Herbal Medicine

Catherine Zollman and Andrew Vickers

Background

The use of plants for healing purposes predates human history and forms the origin of much modern medicine. Many conventional drugs originate from plant sources; a century ago, most of the few effective drugs were plant based. Examples include aspirin (from willow bark), digoxin (from foxglove), quinine (from cinchona bark), and morphine (from the opium poppy). The development of drugs from plants continues, with drug companies engaged in large-scale pharmacological screening of herbs.

Chinese herbalism is the most prevalent of the ancient herbal traditions currently practised in Britain. It is based on concepts of yin and yang and of 'Qi' energy. Chinese herbs are ascribed qualities such as 'cooling' (yin) or 'stimulating' (yang) and used, often in combination, according to the deficiencies or excesses of these qualities in the patient.

Modern Western herbalism emphasizes the effects of herbs on individual body systems. For example, herbs may be used for their

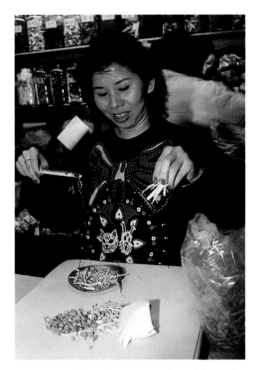

Figure 5.2 Chinese herbalism is the most prevalent of the traditional herbal practices in Britain. Reproduced with permission of Rex Features/ Hafenrichter.

supposed anti-inflammatory, haemostatic, expectorant, antispasmodic, or immunostimulatory properties.

Total out of pocket expenditure on six established complementary therapies in the UK in 1998 was estimated at £450 million with an estimated 20% of the UK population purchasing over the counter herbal remedies. This type of herbal drug use is typically based on a simple matching of a particular herb to particular diseases or symptoms – such as valerian (*Valeriana officinalis*) for sleep disturbance. Originally confined to health food shops, herbal remedies are now marketed in many conventional pharmacies.

Differences from conventional drug use

Although superficially similar, herbal medicine and conventional pharmacotherapy have three important differences.

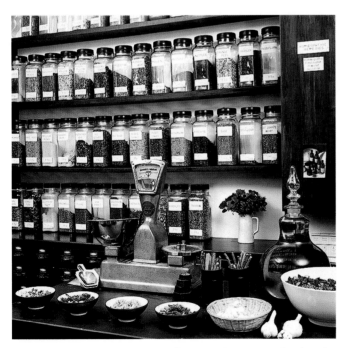

Figure 5.1 Until a century ago most effective medicines were plant based. Reproduced with permission of Paul Biddle/Science Photo library.

Use of whole plants

Herbalists generally use unpurified plant extracts containing several different constituents. They claim that these can work together synergistically so that the effect of the whole herb is greater than the summed effects of its components. They also claim that toxicity is reduced when whole herbs are used instead of isolated active ingredients ('buffering'). Although two samples of a particular herbal drug may contain constituent compounds in different proportions, practitioners claim that this does not generally cause clinical problems. There is some experimental evidence for synergy and buffering in certain whole plant preparations, but how far this is generalizable to all herbal products is not known.

Herb combining

Often, several different herbs are used together. Practitioners say that the principles of synergy and buffering apply to combinations of plants and claim that combining herbs improves efficacy and reduces adverse effects. This contrasts with conventional practice, where polypharmacy is generally avoided whenever possible.

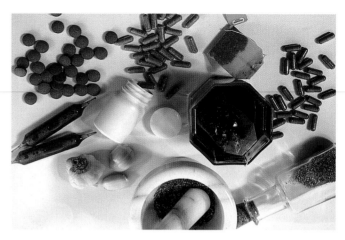

Figure 5.3 Herbal remedies are available in a wide variety of formulations. Reproduced with permission of Alain Dex, Publiphoto Diffusion/Science Photo Library.

> **Box 5.1 Example of a herbal prescription for osteoarthritis**
>
> - Turmeric (*Curcuma langa*) tincture 20 ml: for anti-inflammatory activity and to improve local circulation at affected joints
> - Devil's claw (*Harpagophytum procumbens*) tincture 30 ml: for anti-inflammatory activity and general wellbeing
> - Ginseng (*Panax* spp.) tincture 10 ml: for weakness and exhaustion
> - White willow (*Salix alba*) tincture 20 ml: for anti-inflammatory activity
> - Liquorice (*Glycyrrhiza glabra*) 5 ml: for anti-inflammatory activity and to improve palatability and absorption of herbal medicine
> - Oats (*Avena sativa*) 15 ml: to aid sleep and for general wellbeing

Diagnosis

Herbal practitioners use different diagnostic principles from conventional practitioners. For example, when treating arthritis, they might observe 'underfunctioning of a patient's systems of elimination' and decide that the arthritis results from 'an accumulation of metabolic waste products'. A diuretic, choleretic, or laxative combination of herbs might then be prescribed alongside herbs with anti-inflammatory properties.

What happens during a treatment?

Herbal practitioners take extensive case histories and perform a physical examination. Patients are asked to describe their medical history and current symptoms. Particular attention is paid to the state of everyday processes such as appetite, digestion, urination, defecation, and sleep. Patients are then prescribed individualized combinations of herbs. Some herbal practitioners prepare and dispense their own herbal products. Others use commercially available preparations. Herbal prescriptions are usually made up as tinctures (alcoholic extracts) or teas. Syrups, pills, capsules, ointments, and compresses may also be used. Oral preparations can taste and smell unpleasant.

In addition to the herbal prescription, practitioners may work with their clients to improve diet and other lifestyle factors such as exercise and emotional issues. Follow-up appointments occur after 2–4 weeks. Progress is reviewed and changes made to drugs, doses, or regimen as necessary.

Therapeutic scope

Although herbal preparations are widely used as self-medication for acute conditions, practitioners of herbal medicine tend to concentrate on treating chronic conditions. A typical caseload might include asthma, eczema, premenstrual syndrome, rheumatoid arthritis, migraine, menopausal symptoms, chronic fatigue, and irritable bowel syndrome. Herbalists do not tend to treat acute mental or musculoskeletal disorders.

The aim of herbal treatment is usually to produce persisting improvements in wellbeing. Practitioners often talk in terms of trying to treat the 'underlying cause' of disease and may prescribe herbs aimed at correcting patterns of dysfunction rather than targeting the presenting symptoms. That said, many practitioners prescribe symptomatically as well, such as giving a remedy to aid sleep in a patient with chronic pain.

Research evidence

In laboratory settings, plant extracts have been shown to have a variety of effects, including anti-inflammatory, vasodilatory, antimicrobial, anticonvulsant, sedative, and antipyretic effects. In a typical study, an infusion of lemon grass leaves produced a dose-dependent reduction of experimentally induced hyperalgesia in rats. Given that plants contain pharmacologically active substances, such a finding is not surprising.

Several herbs have been subjected to sufficient research to allow meta-analysis. The best known evidence about a herbal product concerns St John's wort (*Hypericum perforatum*) for treating mild to moderate depression. The herb has generally been found to be significantly superior to placebo and therapeutically equivalent to, but with fewer side effects than, conventional antidepressants.

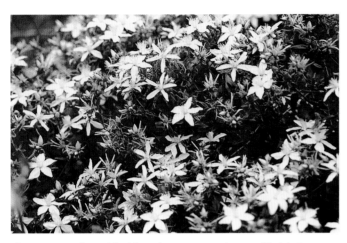

Figure 5.4 A substantial evidence base supports the use of St John's wort for treating mild to moderate depression. Reproduced with permission of Glenis Moore/A-Z Botanical.

Box 5.2 **Key studies of efficacy**

Linde K, Mulrow CD, Berner M, Egger M. St John's wort for depression. *Cochrane Database Syst Rev* 2005; **2**: CD000448.

Hypericum Depression Trial Study Group. Effect of *Hypericum perforatum* (St John's wort) in major depressive disorder: a randomized controlled trial. *JAMA* 2002; **287**(14): 1807–14.

Sheehan MP, Rustin MH, Atherton DJ, *et al*. Efficacy of traditional Chinese herbal therapy in adult atopic dermatitis. *Lancet* 1992; **340**: 13–17.

However, there is still very little evidence on the effectiveness of herbalism as practised – that is, using principles such as combining herbs and unconventional diagnosis. Almost no randomized studies have investigated herbal practitioners treating as they would in everyday clinical work. Perhaps the closest attempt evaluated a traditional Chinese herbal treatment of eczema. As prescriptions depend on patients' exact presentations, only those with widespread, non-exudative eczema were included. Eighty-seven adults and children, refractory to conventional first and second line treatment, were randomized to a crossover study that compared a preparation of about 10 Chinese herbs with a placebo consisting of herbs thought to be ineffective for eczema. Highly significant reductions in eczema scores were associated with active treatment but not with placebo. At long-term follow-up, over half of the adults (12/21) and over 75% of the children (18/23) who continued treatment had a greater than 90% reduction in eczema scores.

Safety

Many plants are highly toxic. Herbal medicine probably presents a greater risk of adverse effects and interactions than any other complementary therapy. There are case reports of serious adverse events after administration of herbal products. In most cases the herbs involved were self-prescribed and bought over the counter or obtained from a source other than a registered practitioner. In the most notorious instance, several women developed rapidly progressive interstitial renal fibrosis after taking Chinese herbs prescribed by a slimming clinic.

As well as their direct pharmacological effects, herbal products may be contaminated, adulterated, or misidentified. Adverse effects seem more common with herbs imported from outside Europe and North America. In general, patients taking herbal preparations regularly should receive careful follow-up and have access to appropriate biochemical monitoring.

As with many complementary therapies, information on the prevalence of adverse effects is limited. Phytonet, a Europe-wide initiative, has begun to operate a type of yellow card system to collect and collate adverse events reported by herbalists. In the UK, the National Poisons Unit has set up a database to record adverse events and interactions, but, without a more systematic reporting scheme, the true incidence of such events will remain unknown. Regulators of conventional medicines, such as the Medicines and Healthcare products Regulatory Authority (MHRA), are becoming more interested in herbal products. The MRHA has produced a report for professionals and advice for the public about the safety of herbal medicines.

Box 5.3 **Sources of information on herbal products**

- National Poisons Information Service: contact details for poisons information centres are available in the *British National Formulary*
- National Institute of Medical Herbalists (NIMH): http://www. nimh. org.uk
- European Scientific Cooperative On Phytotherapy (ESCOP): founded in June 1989 as an umbrella organization representing national phytotherapy associations across Europe to advance the scientific status of phytomedicines and to assist with the harmonization of their regulatory status at the European level. They administer the Phytonet database, http://www.escop.com

Further information
- Continuing professional development paper on herbal interactions from the *Pharmaceutical Journal*: http://www.pjonline.com/pdf/cpd/pj_20030125_herbal10.pdf
- University of Michigan provides a summary of selected drug–herb interactions: http://www.med.umich.edu/1libr/aha/umherb01.htm

---

Interactions of herbal products with conventional drugs have been described. Some well characterized interactions exist, and competent medical herbalists are trained to take a detailed drug history and avoid these. The most common interaction is for herbs to change the metabolism of a conventional drug, reducing its effectiveness. Other interactions are not clearly defined. Problems are more likely to occur with less well qualified practitioners, more unusual combinations of agents, patients taking several conventional drugs, and those who self-prescribe herbal medicines. If patients are taking conventional drugs, herbal preparations should be used with extreme caution and only on the advice of a herbalist who is familiar with the relevant conventional pharmacology.

Table 5.1 Important potential interactions between herbal preparations and conventional drugs.

Herb	Conventional drug	Potential problem
Echinacea used for > 8 weeks	Anabolic steroids, methotrexate, amiodarone, ketoconazole	Hepatotoxicity
Feverfew	Non-steroidal anti-inflammatory drugs	Inhibition of herbal effect
Feverfew, garlic, ginseng, gingko, ginger	Warfarin	Altered prothrombin time/INRI
Ginseng	Phenelzine sulphate	Headache, tremulousness, manic episodes
Ginseng	Oestrogens, corticosteroids	Additive effects
St John's wort	Monoamine oxidase inhibitor and serotonin reuptake inhibitor antidepressants	Mechanism of herbal effect uncertain; insufficient evidence of safety with concomitant use; therefore not advised
Valerian	Barbiturates	Additive effects, excessive sedation
Kyushin, liquorice, plantain, uzara root, hawthorn, ginseng	Digoxin	Interference with pharmacodynamics and drug level monitoring
Evening primrose oil, borage	Anticonvulsants	Lowered seizure threshold
Shankapulshpi (Ayurvedic preparation)	Phenytoin	Reduced drug levels, inhibition of drug effect
Kava	Benzodiazepines	Additive sedative effects, coma
Echinacea, zinc (immunostimulants)	Immunosuppressants (such as corticosteroids, cyclosporin)	Antagonistic effects
St John's wort, saw palmetto	Iron	Tannic acid content of herbs may limit iron absorption
Kelp	Thyroxine	Iodine content of herb may interfere with thyroid replacement
Liquorice	Spironolactone	Antagonism of diuretic effect
Karela, ginseng	Insulin, sulphonylureas, biguanides	Altered glucose concentrations; these herbs should not be prescribed in diabetic patients

Data from Miller (1998).

(a)   (b)

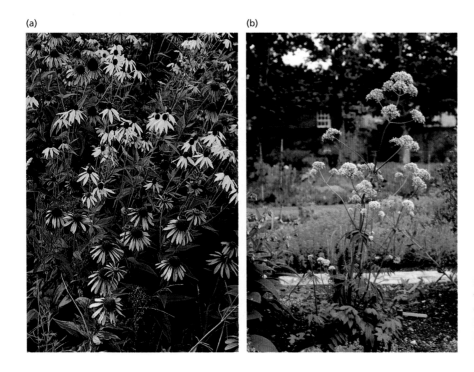

Figure 5.5 Several herbal products interact with conventional drugs – such as Echinacea (a) with anabolic steroids, and valerian (b) with barbiturates. Reproduced with permission of NHPA/Stephen Krasemann (a) and Glenis Moore/A-Z Botanical (b).

Practitioners

Herbalists generally work as sole practitioners or in complementary medicine clinics. Few have conventional healthcare qualifications. There seems to have been little penetration of herbal medicine into the NHS. A small number of doctors practise herbalism, but this is often not integrated into their NHS work. Some ethnic groups have their own indigenous herbal practitioners, such as Hakims or Ayurvedic practitioners from the Indian subcontinent.

Training

There are many different courses in herbalism and substantial variation in the content and standard of teaching. The most comprehensively trained practitioners are known as medical herbalists and are members of the National Institute of Medical Herbalists (NIMH). The NIMH is a professional body and as such is not directly responsible for the academic training of its future members. Schools and universities offering courses in herbal medicine must apply to the board and pass through the accreditation procedure to enable their graduates to become practising members of the NIMH. Training usually includes at least 500 hours of supervised clinical practice and training in nutrition, communication skills, pharmacology, pharmacognosy, botany, pathology, conventional clinical diagnosis, biochemistry, physiology, and research skills. Courses last the equivalent of 4 years full time and lead to BSc degrees in herbal medicine. Each course must reach the minimum standards as set out in the accreditation board's guidelines. Members of the NIMH are invited to a wide variety of postgraduate seminars and a formalized postgraduate continuing professional development scheme is currently being implemented.

Training in Chinese herbalism may be additional to training in acupuncture or may stand on its own. Some British courses involve student placement in China.

Courses in herbal medicine for doctors range from 2-day introductions to 2-year programmes leading to a diploma in herbal medicine.

Regulation

There are a number of professional associations representing the interests of a variety of herbal or traditional medicines in the UK today. The majority of these associations come together under the umbrella of the European Herbal Practitioners Association providing a single voice for the profession.

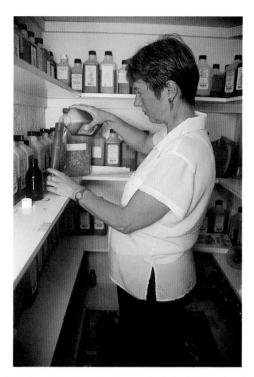

Figure 5.6 Many herbal prescriptions are individually formulated and dispensed by herbal practitioners themselves. Reproduced with permission of BMJ/Ulrike Preuss.

The herbal profession is moving from a system of voluntary to statutory regulation, which should be in place by 2009. A statutory regulator will hold a single register of practitioners who have met minimum standards of training and development, and codes of behaviour and practice.

Regulation of herbal products, however, remains problematic. The constituents of any particular herbal product, such as echinacea or St John's wort, often vary from batch to batch and manufacturer to manufacturer.

Further reading

Brinker F, Stodart N. *Herb Contraindications and Drug Interactions*. Oregon: Eclectic Medical Publications, 1998.

Chan K, Cheung L. *Interactions between Chinese Herbal Medicinal Products and Orthodox Drugs*. London: Taylor and Francis, 2003.

Miller LG. Herbal medicinals: selected clinical considerations focusing on known or potential drug-herb interactions. *Arch Intern Med* 1998; **158:** 2200–11.

Mills S. *The Essential Book of Herbal Medicine*. London: Arkana, 1993.

Mills S, Bone K. *Principles and Practice of Phytotherapy Modern Herbal Medicine*. Edinburgh: Churchill Livingstone, 1999.

Mills S, Bone K. *The Essential Guide to Herbal Safety*. Edinburgh: Churchill Livingstone, 2004.

Newall CA, Anderson LA, Phillipson JD. *Herbal Medicines. A Guide for Healthcare Professionals*. London: Pharmaceutical Press, 1996.

Phil RB. *Herbal–Drug Interactions and Adverse Effects: An Evidence-Based Quick Reference Guide*. New York: McGraw-Hill, 2004.

Box 5.4 **Main regulatory and registering body in herbal medicine**

- European Herbal and Traditional Medicine Practitioners Association: members include organizations representing Ayurveda, Chinese herbal medicine, traditional Tibetan medicine, and Western herbal medicine

  8 Lyon Yard, Tremadoc Road, London, SW4 4NQ, UK. Tel: 020 7627 2680; fax: 020 7627 8947; email: info@ehpa.eu; URL: http://www.ehpa.org.uk

CHAPTER 6

Homeopathy

Catherine Zollman and Andrew Vickers

Background

Homeopaths treat disease using very low dose preparations administered according to the principle that 'like should be cured with like'. Practitioners select a drug that would, if given to a healthy volunteer, cause the presenting symptoms of the patient. For example, the homeopathic remedy *Allium cepa* is derived from the common onion. In a healthy person, contact with raw onions typically causes lacrimation, stinging and irritation around the eyes and nose, and a clear nasal discharge. *Allium cepa* might be prescribed to patients with hay fever, especially if both nose and eyes are affected.

Other common homeopathic medicines include those made from plants such as belladonna, arnica, and chamomile; minerals such as mercury and sulphur; animal products such as sepia (squid ink) and lachesis (snake venom); and, more rarely, biochemical substances such as histamine or human growth factor. The remedies are prepared by a process of serial dilution and succussion (vigorous shaking). The more times this process of dilution and succussion is performed, the greater the 'potency' of the remedy.

Prescribing strategies in homeopathy vary considerably. In what is often termed 'classical homeopathy', practitioners attempt to identify the single medicine that corresponds to a patient's general 'constitution' – a complex picture incorporating current illness, medical history, family history, personality, and behaviour. Two patients with identical conventional diagnoses may receive very different homeopathic medicines.

Other practitioners prescribe combinations of medicines ('complex homeopathy') or prescribe on the basis of conventional diagnosis alone. There is currently insufficient evidence concerning the relative benefits of the different approaches to treatment.

How can homeopathy work?

It is well known that many homeopathic medicines are ultramolecular – that is, they are diluted to such a degree that not even a single molecule of the original solute is likely to be present. As drug actions are conventionally understood in biochemical terms, homeopathy presents an enormous intellectual challenge, if not a complete impasse. Many scientists have suggested that the clinical effects of homeopathic medicines are solely due to the placebo

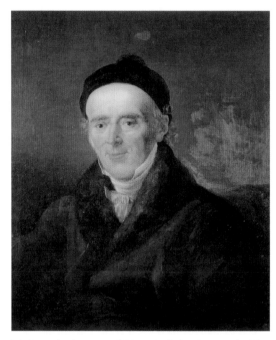

Figure 6.1 Samuel Hahnemann (1755–1843), the German physician who first described homeopathy, began his pioneering experiments in the 1790s. Reproduced with permission of the British Homeopathic Association.

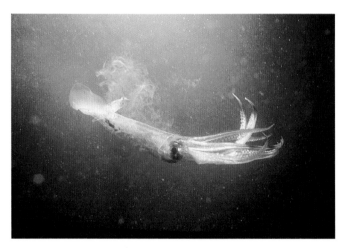

Figure 6.2 Homeopathic medicines are made from various materials, including animal products such as sepia from squid ink. Reproduced with permission of Silvestris.

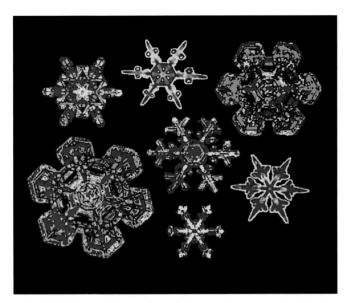

Figure 6.3 The complex lattice formations created by water molecules are thought by some to hold the key to understanding the mechanism by which homeopathy might work. Reproduced with permission of Scott Camazine/ Science Photo Library.

effect. However, there have been rigorous, replicated, double blind, randomized trials, including some *in vitro* studies, showing significant differences between homeopathic and placebo tablets.

The response to this has been mixed. Some people remain unconvinced by the evidence, claiming that there must be another explanation, such as methodological bias, for the results. Others point out that the evidence is very strong and argue that homeopathic medicines must work by some as yet undefined mechanism.

What happens during a treatment?

Consultations by homeopaths for chronic conditions include an extremely detailed case history. Patients are asked to describe their medical history and current symptoms. Particular attention is paid to the 'modalities' of presenting symptoms – that is, whether they change according to the weather, time of day, season, and so on. Information is also gathered about mood and behaviour, likes and dislikes, responses to stress, personality, and reactions to food. The overall aim of the history taking is to build up a 'symptom picture' of the patient. This is matched with a 'drug picture' described in the homeopathic *Materia medica*. On this basis, one or more homeopathic medicines are prescribed, usually in pill form. Sometimes treatment consists of only one or two doses. In other cases a regular daily dose is used.

Two to 6 weeks after the start of treatment, progress is reviewed and alterations made to the remedy or dilution. A patient's initial symptom picture commonly matches more than one homeopathic remedy, and follow-up allows the practitioner to make an empirical judgment on whether a particular remedy was the correct one to prescribe. If the patient is doing well the practitioner may stop treatment and monitor progress. If symptoms recur, the treatment may be repeated at the same or higher potency. If the symptom

Box 6.1 **Examples of drug pictures of commonly prescribed homeopathic medicines**

Aconite (*Aconitum napellus*): shock
- Sudden or violent onset
- Ailments from shock, fright, or fear
- Intense fear; terror stricken; predicts time of death
- Restlessness with fear of death
- Ailments from exposure to cold or dry wind
- Worse with violent emotions, cold, or at night (especially around midnight)
- Better with open air or wine

Chamomile (*Matricaria chamomilla*): teething infant
- Child wants to be carried and is then quieter
- Twitchings and convulsions during teething
- Frantic irritability with intolerance of pain
- Ugly, cross, uncivil, and quarrelsome
- Colic after anger
- Worse with anger, night, dentition, or coffee
- Better with being carried or during warm, wet weather

***Rhus toxicodendron*: joint pains worse with first movement and rest, and better with motion**
- Pain and stiffness worse in damp weather
- Irritability and restlessness at night, driving out of bed
- Back pains and stiffness compelling constant movement in bed
- Urticaria, vesicles; cold air makes skin painful
- Asthma alternating with skin eruptions
- Worse with exposure to wet, cold, before storms, rest, or first movement
- Better with heat, continued motion, rubbing, or hot bath

Modified from Leckridge (1997).

Box 6.2 **Examples of symptomatic homeopathic prescribing**

Remedy	Condition
Cuprum	Leg cramps
Chamomile	Teething
Arnica	Bruising and trauma
Cantharis	Cystitis
Aconite	Croup
Colocynth	Infantile colic
Rhus tox	Joint pain

picture has changed at follow-up, a different homeopathic prescription may be given even though the conventional diagnosis remains unchanged.

Homeopathic consultations in private practice may last over an hour, although many NHS general practitioners practise basic homeopathy in 10–15-minute appointments. Many homeopaths also recommend changes to diet and lifestyle, and some, usually non-medical homeopaths, advise against vaccination (see section on safety below).

Therapeutic scope

Most of a typical homeopath's caseload consists of chronic or recurrent conditions such as eczema, rheumatoid arthritis, fatigue disorders, asthma, migraine, dysmenorrhoea, irritable bowel syndrome, recurrent upper respiratory or urinary tract infections, and mood disorders. Homeopaths also treat a substantial number of patients with ill-defined illness that has not been given a conventional diagnosis. Children are much more commonly treated by homeopaths than by other types of complementary practitioner.

Some homeopaths say that few conditions are truly outside their remit, and the homeopathic case literature includes treatment of complaints as diverse as tuberous sclerosis, infertility, myasthenia gravis, fear of flying, and cystic fibrosis. That said, opinions about what can be effectively treated by homeopathy differ widely, even among homeopaths, with medically trained practitioners generally being more conservative than non-medical ones. It is also used, often by self-prescription, to treat various acute conditions such as the common cold, bruising, hay fever, and joint sprains.

Research evidence

Not all homeopathic medicines are ultramolecular. Some homeopathic gels and ointments contain identifiable amounts of herbal extracts, and there is good evidence that some of these are effective for musculoskeletal pain.

Given the difficulties in understanding how ultramolecular homeopathy may work, researchers have concentrated on establishing whether it is a placebo treatment. A meta-analysis, published in the *Lancet*, examined over 100 randomized, placebo controlled trials and found an odds ratio of 2.45 (95% confidence interval 2.05 to 2.93) in favour of homeopathy. The authors concluded that, even allowing for publication bias, 'the results of our meta-analysis are not compatible with the hypothesis that the clinical effects of homeopathy are completely due to placebo'. Nonetheless, the research base for homeopathy has not importantly progressed since the publication of this meta-analysis and many researchers remain sceptical, especially given the scientific implausibility of homeopathy.

The notorious Benveniste affair, which involved accusations of fraud and scientific misconduct after the publication of an *in vitro* experiment in *Nature*, continues to dampen enthusiasm for basic research in homeopathy. Nonetheless, some currently unreplicated laboratory studies have reported biological effects of homeopathic medicines on animals, plants, and cells – some at ultramolecular dilutions.

Evidence is less clear on the effectiveness of homeopathy as it is generally practised for the conditions that homeopaths usually treat. Many trials have investigated treatment of an acute condition with a single remedy. This makes research easier but does not reflect the real world of homeopathic clinical practice. For example, in the best known UK trial, 144 patients with hay fever were randomized to receive either homeopathically prepared grass pollen or placebo. Though there was a significant result in favour of homeopathy, implications for clinical practice are unclear as most homeopaths do not treat hay fever with homeopathic grass pollen alone.

There is currently insufficient evidence that homeopathy is clearly efficacious for any single clinical condition particularly as few of the existing studies of homeopathy have been independently replicated.

Safety

Serious unexpected adverse effects of homeopathic medicines are rare. 'Aggravation reactions', when symptoms become acutely and transiently worse after starting homeopathic treatment, have been described and are said by homeopaths to be a good prognostic factor.

A potentially more serious issue is the belief of some practitioners that conventional drugs reduce the efficacy of homeopathy. Serious adverse events have resulted from patients failing to take essential conventional treatments while using homeopathy. Some, mainly non-medical, homeopaths are also strongly against vaccination, although the official policy of the Society of Homeopaths is to give patients information and choice and not to pressurize against immunization. Homeopaths may offer alternatives to

---

Box 6.3 **Key studies of efficacy**

Kleijnen J, Knipschild P, ter Riet G. Clinical trials of homoeopathy. *BMJ* 1991; **302**: 316–23.

Linde K, Clausius N, Ramirez G, *et al*. Are the clinical effects of homeopathy placebo effects? A meta-analysis of placebo-controlled trials. *Lancet* 1997; **350**: 834–43.

Shang A, Huwiler-Müntener K, Nartey L, *et al*. Are the clinical effects of homoeopathy placebo effects? Comparative study of placebo-controlled trials of homoeopathy and allopathy. *Lancet* 2005; **366**(9487): 726–32.

van Haselen RA, Fisher PA. A randomized controlled trial comparing topical piroxicam gel with a homeopathic gel in osteoarthritis of the knee. *Rheumatology (Oxford)* 2000; **39**(7): 714–19.

Vickers AJ. Independent replication of pre-clinical research in homeopathy: a systematic review. *Forsch Komplementarmed* 1999; **6**(6): 311–20.

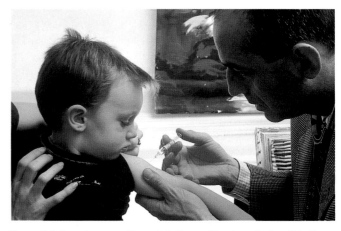

Figure 6.4 Some homeopaths, mainly those without medical qualifications, believe that vaccination does more harm than good. Reproduced with permission of BSIP Laurent & Gille/Science Photo Library.

vaccination. These have not been subjected to clinical trials and cannot therefore be recommended as an effective substitute.

There have been examples of homeopathic medicines being adulterated with drugs, although this is extremely unlikely in the case of registered practitioners in Britain.

Practitioners

About 1000 UK doctors practise homeopathy, although fewer than half of these are full members of the Faculty of Homeopathy. Many are general practitioners who have received only a basic training and who normally prescribe a limited number of remedies for specific acute conditions. More than 2000 homeopaths without a conventional healthcare background are thought to practise in the UK.

In the UK, homeopathy has been part of the NHS since its inception; there are currently five homeopathic hospitals across Scotland and England. The hospitals provide a range of conventional and complementary treatments in addition to homeopathy. Normal NHS conditions apply: patients receive services free at the point of care, and the hospitals are reimbursed through block contracts with health authorities or extracontractual referrals. Some independent homeopaths have had contracts with general practices and Primary Care Trusts to provide treatment for NHS patients.

Homeopathic medicines can be purchased over the counter at chemists and health stores. They can also be prescribed on an FP10 form (GP10 in Scotland) by any doctor registered with the General Medical Council. About 10–20% of the UK population have bought homeopathic products over the counter.

More than 12000 medical doctors and licensed healthcare practitioners administer homeopathic treatment in the UK, France,

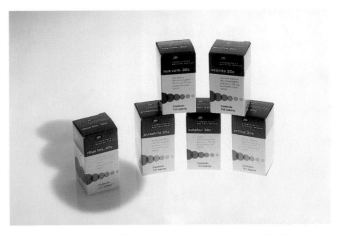

Figure 6.6 A wide range of homeopathic preparations, usually of low potency, are available over the counter. Most are used for self-medication on a simple, symptom matching basis. Reproduced with permission of Boots the Chemist.

and Germany, and homeopathic medicines constitute a substantial share of these countries' over the counter markets.

Training

The Faculty of Homeopathy offers postgraduate courses for statutorily registered healthcare professionals with qualifications recognized in the UK. Students are encouraged to sit the Faculty of Homeopathy's specialist examinations that lead to the recognized qualifications LFHom, MFHom, Vet MFHom, and DFHom. Full membership is available to doctors, nurses, dentists, and veterinary surgeons who have passed the faculty examination.

The minimum entry requirement for the faculty's membership examination (MFHom) is 150–180 hours of study.

Training for homeopaths without a medical background varies. However, the Society of Homeopaths have produced a list of recognized courses, from 3 years full time and 4 years part time. Some training courses lead to university degrees in homeopathy.

Regulation

The Council of Organisations Registering Homeopaths (CORH) is a council of nine current registering bodies for homeopaths

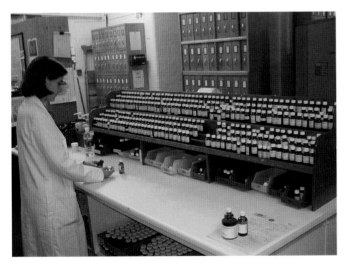

Figure 6.5 The pharmacy of the Royal London Homeopathic Hospital. NHS homeopathic hospitals employ conventionally trained pharmacists, who have additional training in homeopathy and sometimes herbal medicine. They dispense a range of complementary medicines, which are prescribed by medically qualified practitioners. Reproduced with permission of BSIP Laurent & Gille/Science Photo Library.

Box 6.4 Regulatory bodies

- Council of Organisations Registering Homeopaths (CORH)
  Oakwood House, 11 Wingle Tye Road, Burgess Hill, West Sussex RH15 9HR, UK. Tel: 01444 239494; fax: 01444 236848; email: admin@corh.org.uk; URL: http://www.corh.org.uk
- Faculty of Homeopathy: for medically trained homeopaths
  Hahnemann House, 29 Park Street West, Luton LU1 3BE, UK. Tel: 0870 444 3950; fax: 0870 444 3960; URL: http://www.trusthomeopathy.org
- Society of Homeopaths: mainly for non-medically qualified homeopaths
  11 Brookfield, Duncan Close, Moulton Park, Northampton NN3 6WL, UK. Tel: 0845 450 6611; fax: 0845 450 6622; URL: http://www.homeopathy-soh.org

that is working to establish a single UK register for homeopaths who are not on other statutory registers. The Society of Homeopaths is currently the longest established and largest of the professional associations on the council. The Faculty of Homeopaths maintains a register of healthcare professionals who are statutorily registered, including medical homeopaths.

Homeopathy was regulated by the European Union in 2001, by Directive 2001/83/EC.

Further reading

Kayne S. *Homeopathic Pharmacy: theory and practice.* Edinburgh: Churchill Livingstone, 2006.

Leckridge B. *Homoepathy in Primary Care.* Edinburgh: Churchill Livingstone, 1997.

Owen D. *Principles and Practice of Homeopthy.* Oxford: Elsevier Health Sciences UK, 2006.

Swayne J. *The Homoeopathic Method: implications for clinical practice and medical science.* Edinburgh: Churchill Livingstone, 1998.

CHAPTER 7

Hypnosis and Relaxation Therapies

Catherine Zollman, Andrew Vickers, Gill McCall, and Janet Richardson

A wide variety of complementary therapies claim to improve health by producing relaxation. Some use the relaxed state as a means of promoting psychological change. Others incorporate movement, stretches, and breathing exercises. Hypnosis, relaxation, and 'stress management' are found to a certain extent within conventional medicine. They are included here because they are generally not covered in any depth in conventional medical curricula and because they overlap with other, more clearly complementary, therapies. Yoga and meditation are widely available to the general public and are often associated with maintaining fitness and well-being. However, increasingly they are being used therapeutically to alleviate symptoms in chronic and life-limiting conditions. They can also be integrated into health maintenance programmes, for example for older adults and people with depression and anxiety disorders.

Techniques

Hypnosis
Hypnosis is the induction of a deeply relaxed state, with increased suggestibility and suspension of critical faculties. Once in this state, sometimes called a 'hypnotic trance', patients are given therapeutic suggestions to encourage changes in behaviour or relief of symptoms. For example, in a treatment to stop smoking, a hypnosis practitioner might suggest that the patient will no longer find smoking pleasurable or necessary. Hypnosis for a patient with arthritis might include a suggestion that the pain can be turned down like the volume of a radio.

Some practitioners use hypnosis as an aid to psychotherapy. The rationale is that in the hypnotized state the conscious mind presents fewer barriers to effective psychotherapeutic exploration, leading to an increased likelihood of psychological insight.

Relaxation techniques
One well known example of a relaxation technique is known variously as sequential muscle relaxation (SMR), progressive relaxation, and Jacobson relaxation. The subject sits comfortably in a dark, quiet room. He or she then tenses a group of muscles, such as those in the right arm, holds the contraction for 15 seconds, and then releases the muscles while breathing out. After a short rest, this sequence is repeated with another set of muscles. Gradually, different sets of muscle are combined.

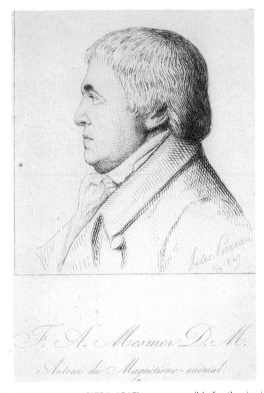

Figure 7.1 Franz Mesmer (1734–1815) was responsible for the rise in popularity, and notoriety, of hypnosis ('mesmerism') in the 18th century.

The Mitchell method involves adopting body positions that are opposite to those associated with anxiety (fingers spread rather than hands clenched, for example). In autogenic training, subjects concentrate on experiencing physical sensations, such as warmth and heaviness, in different parts of their bodies in a learnt sequence. Other methods encourage deepening and slowing the breath and a conscious attempt to let go of tension during exhalation.

Visualization and imagery techniques
These are somewhat akin to hypnosis: the induction of a relaxed state followed by the use of suggestion. In guided imagery, participants are asked to rest back and to listen to a descriptive journey, provided by the facilitator. This might be a walk in the countryside or by the sea, or it might be a more metaphysical journey,

Box 7.1 **Hypnosis techniques that can be employed therapeutically**

Visualization and guided imagery
- Various therapeutic suggestions are made, which alter physiological or emotional response, e.g. 'imagine placing cool, white snow on your eczema and let it absorb the red itchiness ...'

Time distortion
- In hypnotic rehearsal of an invasive procedure, e.g. cannulation or endoscopy, the procedure can be 'happening in the blink of an eye ...'
- For chronic pain, analgesic suggestions followed by 'you are feeling so very comfortable now, that every minute of comfort feels like an hour ...'

Dissociation
- During labour, a woman might be encouraged to 'relax as you watch yourself giving birth ...'

Body dysmorphia
- For patients having chemotherapy, 'you might notice your arm resting beside you as the treatment is dripped into it ...'
- During gynaecological procedures, 'everything below the waist seems to be absorbed into a pool of warm water, so that you float on the surface, and feel nothing below ...'

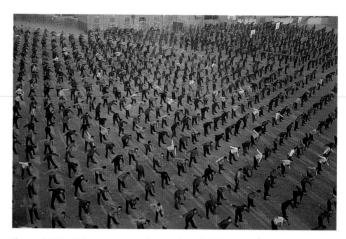

Figure 7.3 In China many people practise tai chi for health promotion on a daily basis.

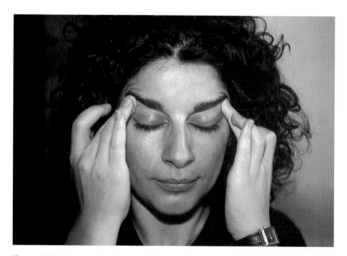

Figure 7.2 Many relaxation techniques aim to increase awareness of areas of chronic unconscious muscle tension. They often involve a conscious attempt to release and relax during exhalation.

for example floating in the clouds. The object of the exercise is to promote a sense of calmness that leads to physical relaxation.

Visualization is a technique where individuals are asked to generate the image themselves. In cancer treatment, for example, some patients may use combative images, for example imagining immune cells as sharks and the cancer cells as small fishes being eaten; another might think of a computer game in which the cancer cells are 'zapped' by spaceships. Others might use more gentle images, such as the sun or water melting or dissolving the cancer away.

Meditation

Many meditative practices date back centuries and have a place in both Western and Eastern cultures. Such practices focus on stilling or emptying the mind. Typically, meditators concentrate on their breath or a sound ('mantra'), which they repeat to themselves. They may, alternatively, attempt to reach a state of 'detached observation' in which they are aware of their environment but do not become involved in thinking about it. In meditation the body remains alert and in an upright position. There are different types of meditation which may or may not be associated with traditional spiritual practices.

Yoga, tai chi, and qigong

Yoga practice involves postures, breathing exercises, and meditation aimed at improving mental and physical functioning. Some practitioners understand yoga in terms of traditional Indian medicine, with the postures improving the flow of 'prana' energy around the body. Others see yoga in more conventional terms of muscle stretching, exercise, and mental relaxation.

Tai chi is a gentle system of exercises originating from China. The best known example is the 'solo form' – a series of slow and graceful movements that follow a set pattern. It is said to improve strength, balance, and mental calmness.

Qigong (pronounced 'chi kung') is another traditional Chinese system of therapeutic exercises. Practitioners teach meditation, physical movements, and breathing exercises to improve the flow of 'Qi', the Chinese term for body energy.

What happens during a treatment?

Hypnosis

In hypnosis, patients normally see practitioners by themselves for a course of hourly or half-hourly treatments. Some general practitioners and other medical specialists use hypnosis as part of their regular clinical work and follow a longer initial consultation with standard 10–15-minute appointments. History taking is used to identify issues and agree on potentially useful suggestions. After an initial relaxation, and often some therapeutic suggestions, patients can also be given a post-hypnotic suggestion that enables them to induce self-hypnosis after the treatment course is completed. Some practitioners undertake group hypnosis, treating up to a dozen

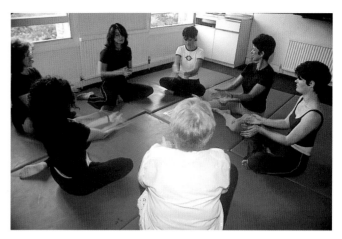

Figure 7.5 Relaxation classes can play a social function in addition to having therapeutic benefits.

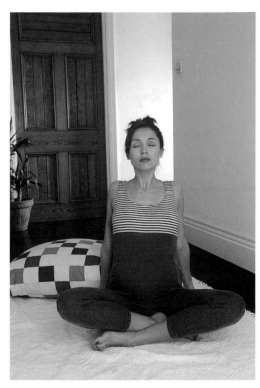

Figure 7.4 Self-hypnosis can be taught to pregnant women as preparation for labour.

patients at a time – for example, teaching self-hypnosis to antenatal groups as preparation for labour.

Relaxation techniques

Most relaxation techniques need to be practised daily. Typically, patients learn a relaxation technique over the course of eight weekly classes, each lasting an hour or so. Between classes, they practise by themselves for 15–30 minutes each day. Some relaxation practices involve elements of imagery and visualization. After the course is over, patients are encouraged to continue on their own, though they may take further classes to learn advanced techniques or to maintain group support. Methods such as sequential muscle relaxation are learnt relatively readily. Relaxation techniques are generally enjoyable, and many healthy individuals practise them without having particular health problems. Relaxation classes can also play a social function.

Unlike in many other complementary therapies, practitioners of relaxation techniques do not make diagnoses. They may use conventional diagnoses as described by the patient to tailor the prescribed programme appropriately. However, in many cases the method of treatment does not depend on a precise diagnosis.

Meditation

As it is primarily a form of internal focusing, meditation can be learnt and practised alone or in groups. Some forms of meditation are taught as a programme, for example mindfulness based stress reduction (MBSR) is traditionally delivered as an 8-week programme in small groups. Weekly sessions typically last for 1 or 1.5 hours. Participants are sometimes given an audiotape to encourage home practice. Meditation retreats over a few days are popular way of deepening the experience. MBSR has, to some extent, been integrated into psychiatry as mindfulness based cognitive therapy (MBCT).

Yoga, tai chi, and qigong

Yoga classes are most often based on a series of postures (Asanas) designed to promote flexibility and strength. Tai chi and qigong are similar but typically involve movements rather than static postures. All three have some overlap with meditation as the attention is very focused. Typically classes last an hour to an hour and a half, and end with a relaxation session. People generally attend classes on an ongoing basis as it takes several years to fully master the techniques.

Yoga therapy is a new discipline that combines traditional yoga with modern medicine and tailors yoga practices to individual clinical needs. Sessions are provided by a yoga therapist to individuals or groups and include physical postures, breathing techniques, and relaxation.

Therapeutic scope

The primary uses of hypnosis and relaxation techniques are in anxiety, disorders with a strong psychological component (such as asthma and irritable bowel syndrome), and conditions that can be modulated by levels of arousal (such as pain and treatment side effects). They are also commonly used in programmes for stress management.

Research evidence

There is good evidence from randomized controlled trials that both hypnosis and relaxation techniques can reduce anxiety, particularly in relation to stressful situations. They are also effective for panic disorders and insomnia, particularly when integrated into a package of cognitive therapy (including, for example, sleep hygiene). A systematic review has found that hypnosis enhances the effects of cognitive behavioural therapy for conditions such as phobia, obesity, and anxiety.

Box 7.3 **Key studies of efficacy**

Eccleston C, Yorke L, Morley S, Williams AC, Mastroyannopoulou K. Psychological therapies for the management of chronic and recurrent pain in children and adolescents. *Cochrane Database Syst Rev* 2003; **1**: CD003968.

Eisenberg DM, Delbanco TL, Berkey CS, *et al.* Cognitive behavioral techniques for hypertension: are they effective? *Ann Intern Med* 1993; **118**: 964–72.

Harvey RF, Hinton RA, Gunary RM, Barry RE. Individual and group hypnotherapy in treatment of refractory irritable bowel syndrome. *Lancet* 1989; **i**: 424–5.

Kirsch I, Montgomery G, Sapirstein G. Hypnosis as an adjunct to cognitive-behavioral psychotherapy: a meta-analysis. *Consult Clin Psychol* 1995; **63**: 214–20.

Ostelo RW, van Tulder MW, Vlaeyen JW, Linton SJ, Morley SJ, Assendelft WJ. Behavioural treatment for chronic low-back pain. *Cochrane Database Syst Rev* 2005; **1**: CD002014.

Randomized controlled trials support the use of various relaxation techniques for treating both acute and chronic pain, although two recent systematic reviews suggest that methodological flaws may compromise the reliability of these findings. Randomized trials have shown hypnosis to be of value in asthma and irritable bowel syndrome. There is evidence from systematic reviews that hypnosis and relaxation techniques are probably not of general benefit in stopping smoking or substance misuse or in treating hypertension.

Relaxation and hypnosis are often used in cancer patients. There is strong evidence from randomized trials of the effectiveness of hypnosis and relaxation for cancer- and procedure-related anxiety and pain, particularly in children, and chemotherapy-induced nausea and vomiting. Some practitioners also claim that hypnosis or relaxation techniques – particularly those incorporating visualization – can prolong life. The preponderance of the evidence, however, is that while such techniques can improve quality of life, they have no effect on survival.

Studies on yoga have generally had similar results to those on other forms of relaxation, and the additional benefits of the exercise component are yet to be clarified. Studies on tai chi suggest that it is a safe form of exercise, even for elderly people or those with rheumatoid arthritis, and has some benefits in terms of balance and mobility.

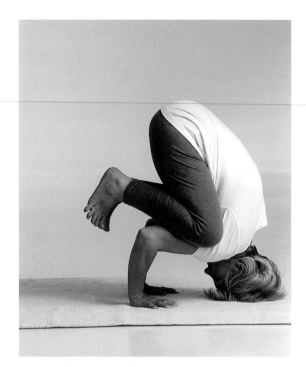

Figure 7.6 Though rare, cases of basilar or vertebral artery occlusion have been reported after certain yoga positions that put stress on the neck.

Safety

Adverse events resulting from relaxation techniques seem to be extremely uncommon. Though rare, there have been reports of basilar or vertebral artery occlusion after yoga postures that put particular strain on the neck. Sequential muscle relaxation should be avoided by people with poorly controlled cardiovascular disease as abdominal tensing can cause the Valsalva response. In patients with a history of psychosis or epilepsy there have been reports of further acute episodes after deep and prolonged meditation.

Hypnosis or deep relaxation, including qigong, can sometimes exacerbate psychological problems – for example, by retraumatising those with post-traumatic disorders or by inducing 'false memories' in psychologically vulnerable individuals. Concerns have also been raised that it can bring on a latent psychosis, although the evidence is inconclusive. Hypnosis should be undertaken only by appropriately trained, experienced, and regulated practitioners. It should be avoided in established or borderline psychosis and personality disorders, and hypnotherapists should be competent at recognizing and referring patients in these states.

Practitioners

Relaxation techniques are often integrated into other healthcare practices. For example, they may be included in programmes of cognitive behavioural therapy in pain clinics or occupational therapy in psychiatric units. Many different complementary therapists, such as osteopaths and massage therapists, may include some relaxation techniques in their work. Some nurses use relaxation techniques in the acute setting, such as in preparation for surgery. A small number of general practices offer regular classes in relaxation, yoga, or tai chi.

Training

The British Society for Medical and Dental Hypnosis (BSMDH) and the British Society of Experimental and Clinical Hypnosis (BSECH) run basic, intermediate, and advanced courses for doctors and other conventionally trained healthcare professionals. Both organizations and the Section of Hypnosis and Psychosomatic Medicine of the Royal Society of Medicine hold regular scientific meetings. There is no standard training in hypnosis for practitioners without a conventional healthcare background.

Box 7.4 **Training and professional organizations**

- The British Society of Clinical and Academic Hypnosis incorporates the British Society for Medical and Dental Hypnosis (BSMDH) founded in 1952/British Society of Experimental and Clinical Hypnosis (BSECH) founded in 1977. National Office 28 Dale Park Gardens, Cookridge, Leeds LS16 7PT, UK. Tel/fax: 0700 056 0309; email: natoffice@bsmdh.com; URL: www.bscah.com
- Royal Society of Medicine, Section on Hypnosis and Psychosomatic Medicine 1 Wimpole Street, London WIN 8AE, UK. Tel: 0207 290 2986; fax: 0207 290 2989; email: hypnosis@roysocmed.ac.uk
- UK Confederation of Hypnotherapy Organisations Suite 401, 302 Regent Street, London W1B 3HH, UK. Tel: 0800 952 0560; URL: http://www.ukcho.co.uk
- British Psychological Society (BPS) St Andrews House, 48 Princess Road East, Leicester LEI 7DR, UK. Tel: 0116 254 9568; fax: 0116 247 0787; URL: http://www.bps.org.uk
- British Association of Counselling and Psychotherapy (BACP) BACP House, 15 St John's Business Park, Lutterworth LE17 4HB, UK. Tel: 0870 443 5252; fax: 0870 443 5161; URL: http://www.bacp.co.uk, http://www.counselling.co.uk
- United Kingdom Council of Psychotherapy (UKCP) 2nd Floor, Edward House, 2 Wakley Street, London EC1V 7LT, UK. Email: info@psychotherapy.org.uk; URL: http://www.ukcp.org.uk
- Centre for Mindfulness Research and Practice Institute for Medical and Social Care Research, Dean Street Building, University of Wales Bangor, Bangor, Gwynedd LL57 1UT, UK. Tel: 0124 838 2939; email: mindfulness@bangor.ac.uk; URL: http://www. bangor.ac.uk/mindfulness
- Yoga Biomedical Trust Royal London Homeopathic Hospital, London WCIN 3HR, UK. Tel: 0207 419 7195; fax: 0207 419 7196; email: yogabio.med@virgin.net; URL: http://www.yogatherapy.org
- British Council for Yoga Therapy email: bcytmembsec@schoolofyoga.co.uk; URL: www.britishcouncilforyogatherapy.org.uk

---

Training in teaching relaxation techniques is provided through various routes from self-teaching, through apprenticeships, to a number of short courses.

A range of training options are available and many yoga centres run courses to train yoga teachers. The Yoga Biomedical Trust also trains yoga therapists, who see patients individually and work on specific health problems.

Regulation

The practice of many relaxation techniques is poorly regulated, and standards of practice and training are variable. This situation is unsatisfactory, but – given the relatively benign nature of many relaxation techniques – this variation in standards usually presents more of a problem of ensuring effective treatment and good professional conduct rather than one of avoiding adverse effects.

For hypnosis and deeper relaxation techniques, poor regulation is a more serious issue. The large number of hypnotherapy registers and the lack of a single regulating body make selecting a practitioner difficult. Hypnotherapists with a conventional healthcare background (such as psychologists, doctors, dentists, and nurses) will be regulated by their conventional professional regulatory bodies. The UK Confederation of Hypnotherapy Organisations (UKCHO), founded in 1998, is an umbrella body for the hypnotherapy profession in the UK which aims to ensure that standards of conduct, ethics, and practice are appropriate for public safety. As a confederation of member organizations, UKCHO does not have any individual members. UKCHO member organizations are either registering bodies and/or accrediting bodies. When hypnosis is used as a psychotherapeutic or psychoanalytical tool, practitioners require appropriate training and experience in clinical psychology, counselling, or psychotherapy. Hypnotherapists who practise in this way should be members of the British Psychological Society, the British Association of Counselling, or the United Kingdom Council of Psychotherapy.

Yoga and meditation are not currently regulated as health interventions. The British Council for Yoga Therapy is currently working with the Prince of Wales's Foundation for Integrated Healthcare to establish a unified, voluntary, self-regulatory structure for all yoga teachers and yoga therapists

Further reading

Barber J. *Hypnosis and Suggestion in the Treatment of Pain: a clinical guide.* New York: W.W. Norton, 1996.

Heap M, Aravind KK. *Hartland's Medical and Dental Hypnosis*, 4th edn. Edinburgh: Churchill Livingstone, 2002.

Kabat-Zinn J. *Full Catastrophe Living.* New York: Delacorte, 1990.

Kabat-Zinn J, Massion MD, Kristeller J, *et al.* Effectiveness of a meditation-based stress-reduction program in the treatment of anxiety disorders. *Am J Psychiatry* 1992; **149**(147): 936–43.

Payne RA. *Relaxation Techniques: a practical handbook for the health care professions.* Edinburgh: Churchill Livingstone, 1995.

Roet B. *Understanding Hypnosis: a practical guide to the health-giving benefits of hypnotherapy and self-hypnosis.* London: Piatkus, 2000.

Rossi EL. *The Psychobiology of Mind–Body Healing: new concepts of therapeutic hypnosis*, revised edn. New York: W.W. Norton, 1993.

Waxman D. *Medical-Dental Hypnosis.* London: Balliere Tindall, 1988.

CHAPTER 8

Manipulative Therapies: Osteopathy and Chiropractic

Catherine Zollman, Andrew Vickers, and Alan Breen

Osteopathy and chiropractic share a common origin in the folk medicine of 19th century America. Between that time and the present they have gradually became recognized as legitimate health professions and since the mid-1980s have been regulated in the UK by general councils established under separate Acts of Parliament (see below). These two professions are commonly referred to as the 'manipulative therapies' (even though other professions use manipulation, and chiropractic and osteopathy use other treatments, such as exercise and education). Nevertheless, they have many similarities, not least a specialist knowledge of manual therapies in the treatment of common musculoskeletal complaints. This chapter will describe their current practise in the UK, where practitioners began to arrive in the early 1900s.

Background

Osteopathy and chiropractic are traditionally 'high street' healthcare professions, making them easy for the public to access. However, access to them through the NHS is problematical, despite their inclusion in the Department of Health's new Musculoskeletal Services Framework.

The main aim of treatment is rehabilitation from disabilities. To pursue this, practitioners first work to rule out underlying health problems with a case history and examination, while at the same time looking for life factors that could interfere with recovery and could be altered by the patient themselves. Then they give an explanation of symptoms, with advice about how to get better, usually accompanied by some kind of manual treatment directed at joints, muscles, and connective tissues.

The best known treatment technique is the 'high velocity thrust': a short, sharp motion usually applied to the spine. This manoeuvre is designed to release structures with a restricted range of movement. High velocity thrusts often produce the sound of joint 'cracking', which is associated with manipulative therapy. There are various methods of delivering a high velocity thrust, depending on where in the body it is being used. Chiropractors have a preference for this kind of manual procedure over repetitive movements, which are often used by osteopaths. However, it is important to state that both professions use both these manual techniques and many more.

Chiropractors and osteopaths, as well as physiotherapists and doctors who have additional training in manipulation, also use a

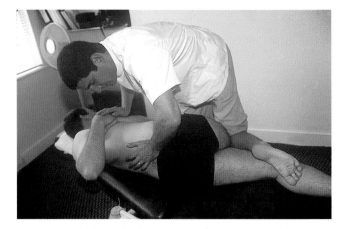

Figure 8.1 The high velocity thrust delivered by a levered thrust is the technique usually used by osteopaths. Reproduced with permission of BMJ/Ulrike Preuss.

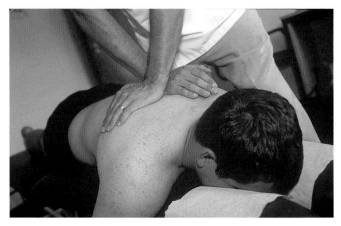

Figure 8.2 The high velocity thrust given as a direct thrust on the spine, as favoured by chiropractors. Reproduced with permission of BMJ/Ulrike Preuss.

range of soft tissue techniques that do not involve joint manipulation. For example, pressure, stretching, and fatiguing of muscles can be used to alter muscle tone or treat spasm. Techniques like these are based on an understanding of subtle neuromuscular behaviour, which conforms to mainstream science. To decide what specific technique to use and how to use it often depends on some finely developed palpatory skills. Some practitioners also have

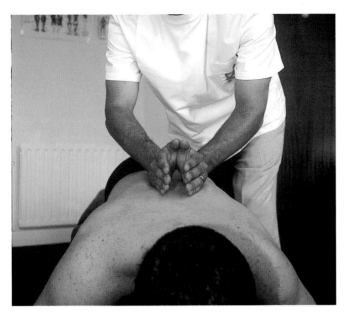

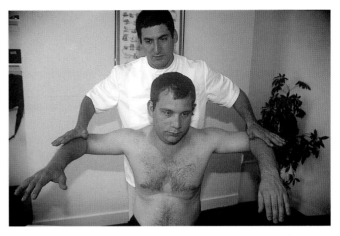

Figure 8.5 Palpatory assessment of areas of muscle spasm and tenderness, restricted joint movements, local differences in skin temperature, and sweat gland activity are all important in making a diagnosis and planning treatment. Reproduced with permission of BMJ/Ulrike Preuss.

Figure 8.3 Chiropractors and osteopaths may use soft tissue techniques to increase a joint's range of movement or to relieve muscular spasm. Reproduced with permission of BMJ/Ulrike Preuss.

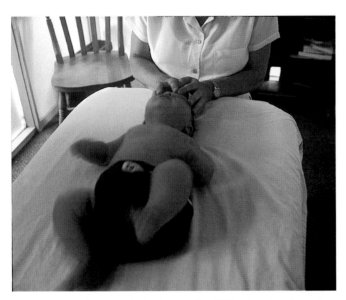

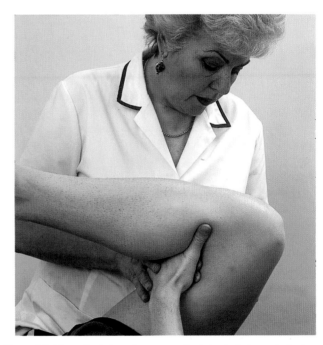

Figure 8.6 Many physiotherapists use manipulative techniques similar to those of chiropractors and osteopaths. Reproduced with permission of Science Photo Library.

Figure 8.4 Cranial osteopathy is often used in children less than 6 months old. The self-limiting nature of many infantile problems (such as colic and irregular sleep patterns) means that evaluation by randomized controlled trials is essential. Reproduced with permission of BMJ/Ulrike Preuss.

sub-specialties, such as cranial osteopathy, craniosacral therapy, or paediatric chiropractic. They also may have preferred techniques that bear the names of their inventors, such as McTimoney and Gonstead. However, with statutory regulation has come the legal requirement to adhere to published standards of proficiency that stipulate the competencies that all must have. Failure to have them can lead to disciplinary proceedings and removal from the respective register. This would be serious for any practitioner, as it is illegal to represent oneself as an osteopath or chiropractor if not on a statutory register.

Recent research has found that attitudes to and techniques for the management of back pain are similar across the chiropractic, osteopathy, and physiotherapy professions. All three recognize the need to promote a return to normal activities and take account of psychological and social factors, but physiotherapists feel more 'connected' to the healthcare system and have a less 'biomedical' approach than chiropractors, who in turn are less likely to endorse a limit on the number of treatment sessions.

What happens during a treatment?

Osteopaths and chiropractors evaluate patients' health status as well as their immediate complaints by taking a history, examining for concurrent health problems, such as high blood pressure, and doing a functional evaluation of the musculoskeletal problem. This involves testing specific ranges of motion and palpating for significant changes in muscle tension. Chiropractors used to X-ray most of their patients to enhance diagnosis, but recent legislation requiring diagnostic radiation to be explicitly justified has reduced this to a minority of patients who have not recovered for specific reasons or need to have serious pathology excluded.

A typical treatment session lasts 15–30 minutes, although first consultations may take longer. A variety of the techniques described above will be used, but sometimes only explanation, reassurance, advice about activity, problem solving, or the prescription of exercise or a follow-up examination may be given at a session. A course of chiropractic or osteopathic treatment for back pain might consist of six sessions, initially frequent to ensure improvement and then at longer intervals to reassess and ensure that the problem is resolving. Osteopaths are more likely than chiropractors to treat on an 'as needed' basis.

Therapeutic scope

Both osteopathy and chiropractic were originally regarded as complete systems of medicine. For example, Andrew Taylor Still, the founder of osteopathy, treated infectious diseases and blindness among a range of conditions. Interestingly, the treatment of back problems features only rarely in his writings. Similarly, early chiropractors believed that most diseases could be attributed to misalignments of the spine and were therefore amenable to treatment with chiropractic. Contemporary practitioners have moved away from this position and concentrate primarily on musculoskeletal disorders. Low back pain is the most common presenting complaint.

There are many guidelines, based on research, on how to manage musculoskeletal disorders. The latest come from the European Commission and cover acute (first 4 weeks), subacute (5–12 weeks), and chronic (over 12 weeks) back pain as well as the prevention of back pain. These are mainly aimed at GPs, and, for the acute and sub-acute stages, recommend excluding pathology, assessing for psychological and social factors, avoiding routine X-rays, and reassessing patients who are not improving. The mainstay of treatment is adequate information and helping the patient to remain active while controlling pain with analgesics (which chiropractors and osteopaths do little of). Manipulation is recommended if the patient is not returning to normal activities. Chronic back pain is more difficult to treat, but exercise, problem-solving advice, and short courses of manipulation are recommended. These largely reflect the approach of the main professions that use manipulation.

Osteopaths and chiropractors also treat neck and shoulder pain, sports injuries, repetitive strain disorders, and headache. These conditions are sometimes associated with osteoarthritis, the progression of which is more likely to be influenced by advice than physical treatment, which is aimed at reducing pain and improving function.

Box 8.1 **Key studies of efficacy**

Systematic reviews

Assendelft WJJ, Morton SC, Yu EI, *et al*. Spinal manipulative therapy for low back pain: a meta-analysis of effectiveness relative to other therapies. *Ann Intern Med* 2003; **138**: 871–81.

Bronfort G, Haas M, Evans RL, *et al*. Efficacy of spinal manipulation and mobilization for low back pain and neck pain: a systematic review and best evidence synthesis. *Spine J* 2004; **4**: 335–56.

European Commission, CBMC. COST B13: European guidelines for the management of low back pain. *Eur Spine J* 2006; **15** (suppl. 2): S125–7.

Gross AR, Hoving JL, Haines TA, *et al*. Manipulation and mobilisation for mechanical neck disorders (review). *Cochrane Library*, 2005.

Rubinstein SM, Peerdeman SM, van Tulder MW, *et al*. A systematic review of the risk factors for cervical artery dissection. *Stroke* 2005; **36**: 1575–80.

Randomized controlled trials

Ferreira ML, Ferreira PH, Latimer J, *et al*. Efficacy of spinal manipulative therapy for low back pain of less than three months' duration. *J Manipulative Physiol Therapeutics* 2003; **26**: 593–601.

Santilli V, Beghi E, Finucci S. Chiropractic manipulation in the treatment of acute back pain and sciatica with disc protrusion: a randomized double-blind clinical trial of active and simulated spinal manipulations. *Spine J* 2006; **6** (2): 131–7.

UK BEAM Trial Team. United Kingdom Back pain Exercise And Manipulation (UK BEAM) randomised trial: effectiveness of physical treatments for back pain in primary care. *BMJ* 2004; 19 November, 1–8.

Research evidence

There is considerable evidence from randomized controlled trials of the effectiveness of spinal manipulation for back and neck pain. However, osteopaths and chiropractors do not treat musculoskeletal pain using manipulation alone, rather as a package of care including advice and exercise. This 'package' has been tested in clinical trials supported by the UK Medical Research Council and Health Technology Assessment Programme. The trial results were published in the *British Medical Journal* in 2004. All three manipulative professions participated, comparing the 'manipulation package of care' with 'best GP' care, which was given by general practitioners who had special additional training in managing back pain. The trial found that the manipulation package, followed by exercise, was moderately better than best GP care at 3 months and slightly better at 12 months. It was also cost-effective and its benefits were not influenced by whether it was given in private (the 'red carpet effect') or NHS premises. None of the 1334 patients in the trial who had manipulation reported any serious adverse effects. Although this evidence reflects only a modest difference, there is a scarcity of specially trained GPs and there is evidence that GPs have difficulty in managing back pain as recommended by guidelines. Manipulative therapy as commonly practised in the UK emerges as a useful approach to back pain, though it is far from a 'magic bullet'.

Around a quarter of the patients who consult chiropractors and osteopaths come for neck pain, and a further 10% for headaches. There is less research evidence about these types of pain than for back pain, especially in relation to lasting effects. The most recent evidence indicates that manual therapy in the form of mobilization may be superior to standard physiotherapy in the short and long term, but there is no evidence that the high velocity type of manipulation is superior to either. There is also little good quality research into the effectiveness of the manipulation package for visceral conditions such as asthma and hypertension, or for any specific manipulative technique.

Safety

Probably the greatest risk from seeing any primary contact health practitioner is that they will fail to detect serious disease. The extent to which this happens in osteopathy and chiropractic is unknown, but around 1% of back pain is associated with such conditions. There is evidence that in chiropractic and osteopathy, around 6% of patients are advised to consult their GPs, most often for hip arthritis or disc prolapse, but very occasionally for a life-threatening illness such as cancer or aortic aneurysm. Another condition that is very rare, but can cause neck pain or headache, is vertebro-basilar arterial dissection – splitting of the wall of one of the arteries, high in the neck, that supplies the brain. This accounts for around 2% of all strokes, reportedly occurring in one per 25 000 adults per year in the UK. If a patient with this condition consults a practitioner for neck pain or headache and it subsequently progresses to a full-blown stroke, it is difficult to know what triggered it. Careful history taking can sometimes alert the practitioner to its presence. However, its seriousness, despite its rarity, has led to a lot of research about whether manipulation could be such a trigger. This research is ongoing, but so far the evidence is inconclusive.

There are other contraindications to manipulation (listed below), and guidelines have been developed that alert practitioners to their nature. However, the commonest adverse effect is a temporary worsening of symptoms. This happens in about half of patients who receive manipulation, is seldom severe, and usually resolves within 24 hours. It is not related to how much the condition ultimately improves. Practitioners have to be alert to presenting symptoms that are already worsening, so that severe 'reactions' can be avoided. In general, practitioners are trained to screen patients and to assess individual risk factors. Even when some techniques, such as high velocity thrusts, are contraindicated, other manipulative treatments may be safe.

Practitioners

Osteopathy and chiropractic are almost exclusively private and based in the community. Many practitioners work alone, often from converted rooms in their own homes. Others work in group clinics, in multidisciplinary practices, or in general practices. Some independent manipulative practitioners have established contracts with general practices or Primary Care Trusts. Most private health insurance schemes now offer some cover for manipulative treatment.

Training

Manual therapies take a long time to learn when combined with training for primary contact healthcare practice. Therefore, most osteopaths take a 4-year, full-time course leading to a BSc degree (BOst). All chiropractors undertake 4–5 years of full-time or mixed-mode training, leading to either BSc honours or masters degrees.

Box 8.2 **Contraindications to high velocity thrusts**

Absolute	Relative	No contraindication
Acute inflammatory arthropathies	Spondylolisthesis with ongoing slippage	Subacute inflammatory arthropathies
Acute fracture or dislocation	Articular hypermobility	Osteoarthritis
Ligament rupture and instability	Post-surgical joints with clinical signs of acute	Spondylolisthesis with no change in slippage
Unstable odontoid peg	inflammation or instability	Post-surgical joints with no signs of instability
Infection	Demineralization	
Vertebro-basilar arterial insufficiency	Benign bone tumours	Acute injuries of soft and bony tissues
Aneurysm	Anticoagulants	Scoliosis
Acute myelopathy		
Acute cauda equina syndrome		

Based on the Mercy guidelines from the Proceedings of the Mercy Center Consensus Conference, Burlingham CA, USA, 1992.

Box 8.3 **Training and educational organizations**

- British Institute of Musculoskeletal Medicine
  PO Box 1116, Bushey, Hertfordshire WD23 9BY, UK. Tel: 0208 421 9910; fax: 0208 386 4183; email: deena@bimm.org.uk; URL: http://www.bimm.org.uk
- London College of Osteopathic Medicine
  8–10 Boston Place, London NW1 6QH, UK. Tel: 0207 262 5250; fax: 0207 723 7492
- Society of Orthopaedic Medicine
  PO Box 223, Patchway, Bristol BS32 4XD, UK. Tel/fax: 0145 461 0255; URL: http://www.somed.org

---

Biological and clinical sciences form a substantial component of all these training courses. Sometimes chiropractors are referred to as 'doctors of chiropractic'.

Many courses in osteopathy and chiropractic are provided by universities. Several organizations run training courses in manipulative techniques specifically for conventional healthcare practitioners. The Manipulative Association of Chartered Physiotherapists runs and accredits postgraduate training in manipulation for physiotherapists. The British Institute of Musculoskeletal Medicine runs courses for medically qualified practitioners but is not a regulatory body. The London College of Osteopathic Medicine organizes a 1-year, full-time osteopathic training course for registered medical practitioners.

Regulation

Osteopathy and chiropractic are the only two complementary health professions that are currently regulated by statute. Two Acts of Parliament passed in the mid-1990s established the General Osteopathic Council and the General Chiropractic Council, UK-wide bodies with statutory powers to register osteopaths and chiropractors. These organizations operate in a similar way to the General Medical Council and have the authority to remove practitioners from the register in disciplinary hearings.

Further reading

Burn L. *A Manual of Medical Manipulation.* Newbury: Petroc Press, 1994.
DiGiovanna EL, Schiowitz S, Dowling D. *An Osteopathic Approach to Diagnosis and Treatment.* Plymouth: Lippincott Raven, 2004.
Haldeman S, ed. *Principles and Practice of Chiropractic,* 3rd edn. London: McGraw Hill, 2005.
Wilson F, ed. *Chiropractic in Europe. An illustrated history.* Leicester: Matador, 2007.
Parsons J, Marcer N. *Osteopathy: models for diagnosis, treatment and practice.* Edinburgh: Churchill Livingstone, 2005.

CHAPTER 9

Massage Therapies

Catherine Zollman, Andrew Vickers, Sheila Dane, and Ian Brownhill

Therapeutic massage is the manipulation of the soft tissue of whole body areas to bring about generalized improvements in health, such as relaxation or improved sleep, or specific physical benefits, such as relief of muscular aches and pains.

Background

Almost all cultures have developed systems of therapeutic massage. Massage techniques play an important part in traditional Chinese and Indian medical care. European massage was systematized in the early 19th century by Per Hendrik Ling, who developed what is now known as Swedish massage.

Ling believed that vigorous massage could bring about healing by improving the circulation of the blood and lymph. In the past 20–30 years, complementary therapists have adapted Swedish massage so as to place greater emphasis on the psychological and spiritual aspects of treatment. Benefits of massage are now described more in terms such as 'calmness' or 'wholeness' than in terms of loosening stiff joints or improving blood flow. In contrast to the vigorous and standardized treatment recommended by Ling, current massage techniques are more gentle, calming, flowing, and intuitive.

Several techniques derive from traditions separate from European massage. In reflexology, areas of the foot are believed to correspond to the organs or structures of the body. Damage or disease in an organ is reflected in the corresponding region, or 'reflex zone' of the foot. When this is palpated the patient is said to experience pain or pricking, no matter how gently pressure is applied. Reflexology treatment consists of massage of the disordered reflex zones.

In aromatherapy, oils derived from plants (essential oils) are added to a base massage oil, which acts as a lubricant during treatment. Although often used purely for their smell, the oils are claimed to have a wide range of medicinal properties, including effects on wound healing, infection, blood circulation, and digestion. They are said to act both pharmacologically, by absorption into the blood through the skin, and by olfactory stimulation. Many massage practitioners use essential oils without claiming to be practising aromatherapy.

Various other complementary disciplines are primarily touch based or have a substantial touch component.

Box 9.1 Examples of other predominantly touch-based therapies

- *Rolfing, structural integration, Hellerwork* – treatments that use deep pressure massage to improve the function of the muscular system
- *Alexander technique, Feldenkrais* – educational systems incorporating exercises and hands-on therapy designed to improve posture, movement, and function
- *Bioenergetics* – massage to aid the psychotherapeutic process
- *'Bodywork'* – any combination of the above

What happens during a treatment?

Massage treatment takes a variety of forms and may last anywhere between 15 and 90 minutes. Treatment follows a case history, which is usually relatively short compared with other complementary therapies but which varies in length depending on the patient's condition and the indications for massage. While giving a standard massage, practitioners will also gather palpatory information, which helps tailor treatment to individual needs. For example, a practitioner will devote extra time to massage an area of increased muscle tension.

The patient is ideally treated unclothed, on a specially designed massage couch. This normally incorporates soft but firm padding and a hole for the face. The treatment room is kept warm and quiet. Soft music may sometimes be played. Practitioners generally treat the whole body, using oil to help their hands move over the patient's body. A variety of strokes are used, including effleurage, petrissage, kneading, and friction. Massage practitioners who treat sports injuries and musculoskeletal disorders may incorporate techniques derived from physiotherapy, osteopathy, and chiropractic. These include deep massage, passive and active stretching, and muscle energy techniques (in which the patient moves against resistance from the practitioner).

Massage can be adapted to the constraints of conventional health settings by limiting work to the head, hands, feet, or back or even by giving a neck and shoulder rub through clothes with the patient sitting in a chair.

Patients usually find massage to be a deeply relaxing and pleasurable experience. Some techniques include strong pressure, which can cause painful sensations, but these are usually short lived.

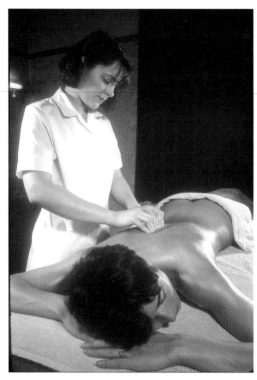

Figure 9.1 A typical massage treatment session. Reproduced with permission of Damien Lovegrove/Science Photo Library.

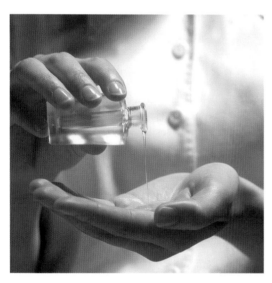

Figure 9.2 UK massage practitioners usually use an oil such as sweet almond oil as a lubricant. Elsewhere in Europe, soap or talcum powder are sometimes used instead. Reproduced with permission of Damien Lovegrove/Science Photo Library.

Box 9.2 **Techniques used in massage**

- *Effleurage* – gentle stroking along the length of a muscle
- *Petrissage* – pressure applied across the width of a muscle
- *Friction* – deep massage applied by circular motions of the thumbs or fingertips
- *Kneading* – squeezing across the width of a muscle
- *Tapotement* – light slaps or karate chops

Therapeutic scope

Massage is mainly used to promote relaxation, treat painful muscular conditions, and reduce anxiety (often described in terms of 'relief from stress'). Practitioners also claim to bring about short-term improvements in sleep disorders and pain, conditions known to be exacerbated by anxiety; massage is widely used for these conditions.

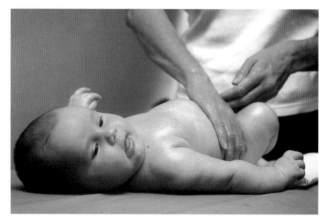

Figure 9.3 Baby massage is one way of encouraging physical interaction and stimulating the developing relationship between parent and child. Reproduced with permission of BMJ/Ulrike Preuss.

Massage is also claimed to have more global effects on health. Practitioners and patients report that massage improves self-image in conditions such as physical disabilities and terminal illnesses. This may result in part from the feelings of general wellbeing that are commonly reported after massage. Touch itself is likely to be therapeutic, particularly in those with limited opportunities for physical contact, such as patients without intimate friends or family or with painful physical conditions.

Massage has also been said to help patients feel cared for. Patients may be more ready to discuss and deal with difficult psychological issues once they are less anxious, feel better about themselves, and have come to trust their care providers. Practitioners say that this is one of the reasons why massage can be an important stepping stone to effective counselling, for example in managing mental health problems or addiction.

Massage has been used to foster communication and relationships in several other settings. Some midwives run 'baby massage' groups where new mothers are taught massage as a means of improving their relationship with their children. In work with children with profound disabilities, where touch may be a primary means of communication, massage techniques have been incorporated into the everyday activities of care workers. Similarly, massage has been used as a way of promoting bonding with premature or unwell babies in special care baby units.

Practitioners of reflexology claim that, in addition to the relaxation and non-specific effects of massage, they can bring about more specific changes in health. One classic reflexology text, for example, includes case histories of ataxia, osteoarthritis, and epilepsy. Similarly, some aromatherapists report benefits in conditions as diverse as infertility, acne, diabetes, and hay fever.

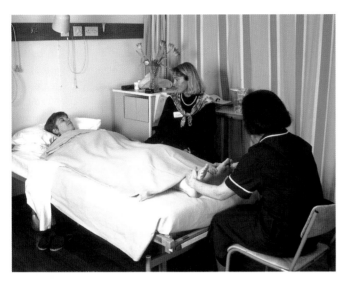

Figure 9.4 Massage on a hospital ward: foot massage has been shown to reduce anxiety even in highly stressful settings. Reproduced with permission of the Royal London Homeopathic Hospital.

Research evidence

To date, most of the clinical trials of massage have focused on psychological outcomes of treatment. Good evidence from randomized trials indicates that massage reduces anxiety scores in the short term in settings as varied as intensive care, psychiatric institutions, hospices, and occupational health. There is more limited evidence that these anxiety reductions are cumulative over time. A Cochrane review of aromatherapy and massage concluded that 'massage and aromatherapy confer short term benefits on psychological well-being, with the effect on anxiety supported by limited evidence'. Practitioners claim that giving patients a concrete experience of relaxation through massage can facilitate their use of self-help relaxation techniques. This has yet to be evaluated.

Box 9.3 Key studies of efficacy

Dale A, Cornwell S. The role of lavender oil in relieving perineal discomfort following childbirth: a blind randomized clinical trial. *J Adv Nurs* 1994; **19**(1): 89–96.

Fellowes D, Barnes K, Wilkinson S. Aromatherapy and massage for symptom relief in patients with cancer. *Cochrane Database of Syst Rev* 2004; **3**: CD002287.

Field T, Morrow C, Valdeon C, Larson S, Kuhn C, Schanberg S. Massage reduces anxiety in child and adolescent psychiatric patients. *Am Acad Child Adolesc Psychiatry* 1992; **31**: 125–31.

Perlman AI, Sabina A, Williams AL, Njike VY, Katz DL. Massage therapy for osteoarthritis of the knee: a randomized controlled trial. *Arch Intern Med* 2006; **166**(22): 2533–8.

Vickers A, Ohlsson A, Lacy JB, Horsley A. Massage therapy for premature and/or low birth-weight infants to improve weight gain and/or to decrease hospital length of stay. *Cochrane Database Syst Rev* 2004; **2**: CD000390.

Williamson J, White A, Hart A, Ernst E. Randomised controlled trial of reflexology for menopausal symptoms. *Br J Obstet Gynaecol* 2002; **109**(9): 1050–5.

Massage also appears to be effective for the treatment of pain. In some cases, such as short-term relief of pain in cancer patients, this appears to be secondary to reduced anxiety. However, there are also trials suggesting that massage is of benefit for conditions such as osteoarthritis or back pain, and that benefits last for many weeks after a course of treatment. This lends support to some of the 'traditional' benefits of massage, such as decreased muscle tension and improved circulation.

Randomized trials have provided some evidence that massage in premature infants is associated with objective outcomes such as more rapid weight gain and development. Many other anecdotal benefits of massage are more subtle and have not been subjected to randomized controlled trials.

There are a limited number of clinical trials examining whether massage techniques such as reflexology or aromatherapy can have specific effects on conditions such as wound healing, irritable bowel syndrome, asthma, or menopausal symptoms. Such trials have generally failed to find any effects specific to aromatherapy oils or reflexology treatment.

Safety

Most massage techniques have a low risk of adverse effects. Cases reported in the literature are extremely rare and have usually involved techniques that are unusual in the UK, such as extremely vigorous massage.

Contraindications to massage are based largely on common sense (for example, avoiding friction on burns or massage in a limb with deep vein thrombosis) rather than empirical data. Massage after myocardial infarction is controversial, although studies have shown that gentle massage is only a moderate physiological stimulus that does not cause undue strain on the heart. There is no evidence that massage in patients with cancer increases metastatic spread, although direct firm pressure over sites of active tumour should generally be avoided.

Considerable concern has been raised about the safety of the oils used in aromatherapy. Although essential oils are pharmacologically active, and in some cases potentially carcinogenic in high concentrations, adverse events directly attributable to them are extremely rare. This may be because in practice the oils are used externally and in low doses (concentrations of 1–3%). However, the lack of a formal reporting scheme for adverse events in aromatherapy means that the safety of essential oils has not been conclusively established and caution is therefore advised.

Massage obviously involves close physical contact. To minimize the risks of unprofessional behaviour in this situation, patients should ensure that practitioners are registered with an appropriate regulatory body.

Practitioners

Like many complementary therapies, massage is usually practised in private in the community. It is also found in conventional health settings, in particular in hospices and in units for learning disability and mental disorders. Massage in these settings is often practised by nurses or by unpaid practitioner volunteers, and much practice

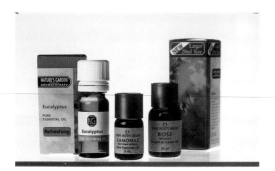

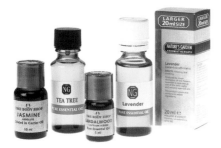

Figure 9.5 More research is needed on both the therapeutic benefits and the safety implications of using essential oils in massage. However, the doses used are low, and problems seem to be extremely rare. Reproduced with permission of Steve Horrel/Science Photo Library.

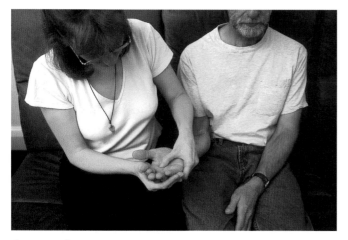

Figure 9.6 If necessary, massage can be adapted to the constraints of conventional healthcare settings by limiting work to the hands, head, or neck and shoulders. Reproduced with permission of BMJ/Ulrike Preuss.

is informal, such as a head and neck rub for a distressed patient. However, an increasing number of professional massage practitioners are now employed in NHS hospitals and general practices.

Training

The variety of training courses is enormous, with many specifically aimed at conventional healthcare workers such as nurses. A central examinations agency, the International Therapy Examinations Council (ITEC), holds examinations in massage and related therapies that are accepted by many organizations. Other courses range from weekend courses in basic massage to university degree courses in therapeutic massage.

Regulation

Practitioners of massage therapies are currently registered by many different professional organizations, a situation that is confusing for those trying to find a reputable practitioner. There are emerging voluntary, self-regulatory bodies for aromatherapy, massage therapy, and reflexology involving the different professional associations. It is probably wise to choose a practitioner from an organization that is a member association of the appropriate emerging regulatory body until the register of practitioners for that profession is established.

Box 9.4 **Voluntary, self-regulatory bodies for massage-based therapies**

- General Council for Massage Therapy, 27 Old Gloucester Street, London WC1N 3XX, UK. Tel: 0870 850 4452; URL: http://www.gcmt.org.uk
- Aromatherapy Council: set up to keep a register of aromatherapists who meet the agreed national standards for their training, professional skills, behaviour, and health; URL: http://www.aromatherapycouncil.co.uk
- Reflexology Forum, Dalton House, 60 Windsor Avenue, London SW19 2RR, UK. Tel: 0800 037 0130; URL: http://www.reflexologyforum.org

Conventional healthcare professionals, who may have undertaken massage training but do not have formal qualifications, are regulated by their own professional body.

Further reading

Holey F, Cook E. *Evidence-Based Therapeutic Massage*. Edinburgh: Churchill Livingstone, 2003.

Mackereth P, Carter A. *Massage and Bodywork: adapting therapies for cancer care*. Edinburgh: Churchill Livingstone, 2006.

Vickers A. *Massage and Aromatherapy: a guide for health professionals*. Cheltenham: Stanley Thomes, 1998.

CHAPTER 10

Unconventional Approaches to Nutritional Medicine

Catherine Zollman, Andrew Vickers, Sheila Dane, Kate Neil, and Ian Brownhill

Although nutrition, as a science, has always been part of conventional medicine, doctors are not taught, and therefore do not practise, much in the way of nutritional therapeutics. Dieticians in conventional settings tend to work mainly with particular patient groups – such as those with diabetes, obesity, digestive or swallowing problems, or cardiovascular risk factors. Apart from the treatment of gross nutritional deficiencies and rare metabolic disorders, other nutritional interventions generally fall outside the mainstream and can therefore be described as complementary medicine. (However, note that unconventional approaches to weight loss will not be covered in this chapter.)

Background

There is a wide spectrum of complementary nutritional practices. These range from specific, well researched, biochemically understood treatments that are provided by well trained practitioners to unresearched, biochemically implausible interventions popularized by spectacular claims in the lay press and largely used without professional supervision.

Just which treatments are 'conventional' and which are 'complementary' is subject to debate. Some, such as fish oil supplements for patients with rheumatoid arthritis, have many of the features of a conventional medical treatment – a biochemical mechanism and support from randomized trials – but are, nonetheless, often considered unconventional. Other interventions were originally considered complementary but are now part of conventional practice. Probably the best example is the high fibre diet, rich in fruit and vegetables. 'Alternative' practitioners of the 19th century, such as John Kellogg, advocated such a diet at a time when conventional nutritional authorities tended to see meat and potatoes as the best food, even to the extent of denigrating the importance of vegetables and describing wheat bran as 'refuse'.

Nutritional interventions

Unconventional nutritional interventions can be broadly divided into three categories: nutritional supplements, dietary modification, and therapeutic systems.

Nutritional supplements

As well as various vitamins and minerals, the range of nutritional supplements includes many animal and plant products. Some of these have known active ingredients, such as γ-linolenic acid in evening primrose oil. Others, such as blue-green algae and kelp, have not been fully characterized biochemically. Some supplements are taken to improve general health and performance, while others are for specific clinical indications. Most are taken in pill form. There is some overlap between herbal and nutritional supplements.

Box 10.1 **Examples of nutritional supplementation**

- High dose vitamin C for cancer
- Zinc for the common cold
- High dose vitamins for learning disability ('orthomolecular' therapy)
- Evening primrose oil for atopic dermatitis
- Evening primrose oil for premenstrual syndrome
- Vitamin B$_6$ for morning sickness
- Vitamin B$_6$ for premenstrual syndrome
- Garlic for lowering cardiovascular risk
- Multivitamins for improvement in general health

Dietary modification

This involves more comprehensive changes in eating patterns. Many diets, such as vegetarianism and veganism, originated as

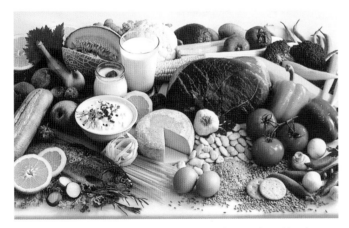

Figure 10.1 Conventional doctors only rarely make use of nutritional interventions, which is perhaps one reason why nutritional medicine has come to be regarded as part of complementary medicine.

'movements' characterized by political and ecological concerns, a moral stance towards food, and a view of diet as inseparable from lifestyle. Many diets are based on theoretical considerations rather than empirical data. For example, the rationale for the Hay diet's principle that starch and protein should not be eaten together is that each type of food requires a different pH for optimum digestion. The principle of the Stone Age diet is that humans are not adapted by evolution to eat grains and pulses.

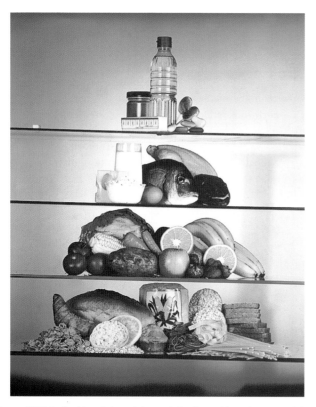

Figure 10.2 In the Hay diet, proteins and starch must be eaten separately, though fruit and vegetables can be eaten with either.

Box 10.2 **Examples of diets claimed to improve general health**

- *Hay diet* – proteins and carbohydrates are eaten separately
- *Blood type diet* – an ideal diet should be determined by an individual's inherited ABO blood type
- *Raw foods diet* – avoids cooked foods
- *Stone Age diet* – avoids grains, pulses, and other products of the agricultural revolution
- *Macrobiotic diet* – largely based on grains and vegetables. Foods are chosen and balanced in accordance with traditional oriental principles such as yin and yang
- *Veganism* – avoids all animal products

Therapeutic systems

These include techniques such as elimination dieting and naturopathy. Elimination dieting is based on the principle that foods particular to each patient may contribute to chronic symptoms or disease when eaten in normal quantities. Unlike classic allergy, these 'food intolerances' do not involve a conventionally understood immune mechanism nor do they inevitably have a rapid onset. Diagnosis consists of eliminating all but a few foods from the diet and then reintroducing foods one by one to see if they provoke symptoms. After a period of complete exclusion, the problem substances can usually be gradually reintroduced without recurrence of symptoms. Although practitioners commonly diagnose wheat and dairy 'intolerance', each patient is said to be sensitive to a different set of foods.

Naturopathy is a therapeutic system emphasising the philosophy of 'nature cure' and incorporating dietary intervention among other practices such as hydrotherapy and exercise. For example, a naturopath might advise a patient with recurrent vaginal candidiasis to undertake a limited fast, to reduce the intake of foods containing sugar and yeast, and to take herbal and probiotic preparations.

Another therapeutic system tests patients for 'subclinical' nutritional deficiencies – thought to arise where systems of food

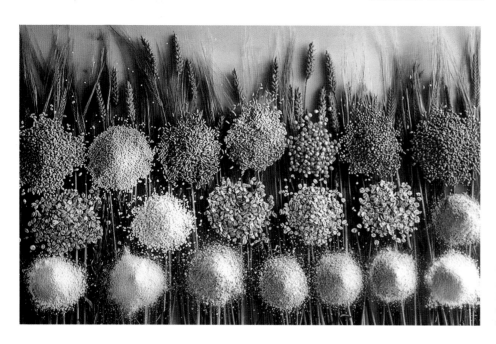

Figure 10.3 In the Stone Age diet, grains, pulses, and other products of the agricultural revolution must be avoided. Such exclusion diets can be highly restrictive, socially disruptive, and expensive.

intake, digestion, or absorption are not fully functional – and gives appropriate supplementation.

What happens during a treatment?

Many people make unconventional nutritional changes without consulting a practitioner (see below). Where practitioners are involved in treatment, consultations may involve some form of testing for deficiencies of particular nutrients or hidden allergies. Such tests include biochemical assays of the vitamin and mineral content of blood or hair. In 'Vega' or electrodermal testing, an electric circuit is made that includes both the patient and the food-stuff suspected of causing disease. Electrical readings are said to confirm or refute the particular foodstuff's involvement. In applied kinesiology, practitioners claim to be able to diagnose an allergy or deficiency on the basis of changes in muscle function.

Evidence of therapeutic scope

There is evidence that exclusion dieting can be of benefit for various conditions including rheumatoid arthritis, hyperactivity, and migraine. However, only a minority of patients with such conditions seem to benefit, and it is not yet possible to select these patients in advance. Randomized trials have shown that increasing the consumption of polyunsaturated fatty acids – for example, by supplementation with products such as fish oils or evening prim-rose oil – and reducing saturates can be beneficial in hypertriglyc-eridaemia, rheumatoid arthritis, and inflammatory bowel disease.

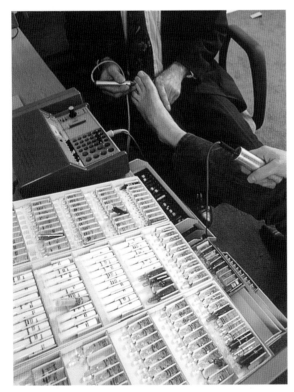

Figure 10.4 Vega testing is said to identify patients' individual food intolerances. Although its validity remains uncertain, it is often used to draw up personalized elimination diet programmes.

Box 10.4 **Key studies of efficacy or reliability**

Caraballoso M, Sacristan M, Serra C, Bonfill X. Drugs for preventing lung cancer in healthy people. *Cochrane Database Syst Rev* 2008; **1**: CD002141.

Douglas RM, Hemilä H, Chalker E, Treacy B. Vitamin C for preventing and treating the common cold. *Cochrane Database Syst Rev* 2007; **3**: CD000980.

Fortin PR, Lew RA, Liang MH, *et al*. Validation of a meta-analysis: the effects of fish oil in rheumatoid arthritis. *J Clin Epidemiol* 1995; **48**: 1379–90.

Malouf R, Grimley Evans J, Areosa Sastre A. Folic acid with or without vitamin B12 for cognition and dementia. *Cochrane Database Syst Rev* 2007; **3**: CD004514.

Schmidt MH, Mocks P, Lay B, *et al*. Does oligo antigenic diet influence hyperactive/conduct-disordered children – a controlled trial. *Eur Child Adolesc Psychiatry* 1997; **6**: 88–95.

Sethi TJ, Kemeny DM, Tobin S, Lessof MH, Lambourn E, Bradley A. How reliable are commercial allergy tests? *Lancet* 1987; **i**: 92–4.

The evidence for most other unconventional nutritional interventions in treating disease is generally either negative or non-existent. For example, randomized trials have failed to show any benefit from high dose vitamin C for cancer; megadose therapy for Down's syndrome, learning disability, or schizophrenia; the Dong diet for arthritis; essential fatty acid supplementation for psoriasis or premenstrual syndrome; or vitamin B_6 for carpal tunnel syndrome. Supplementation has been found to be ineffective (or even harmful) for cancer prevention, heart disease, arthritis, and cognitive impairment in elderly people.

Many unconventional diets are claimed to have benefits in specific conditions and general effects on physical health, mental wellbeing, and even spiritual development. Apart from those discussed above, these have not been evaluated systematically. There has been no rigorous research on the naturopathic approach to chronic disease or on individualized nutritional therapy.

Nutritional tests

While some unconventional laboratories use assays and methods of quality control similar to those used in mainstream biochemical laboratories, others may be less reliable. In studies where duplicate samples of hair or blood were sent to 'alternative' nutritional testing laboratories there was low agreement in results for the same individual. In one investigation several laboratories that advertise services to the general public failed to report fish allergy in subjects who were allergic to fish but ascribed numerous (but inconsistent) allergies to healthy controls. Studies have also found that practitioners of techniques such as applied kinesiology are unable to obtain consistent results from duplicate blinded samples.

Safety

Most unconventional diets recommend generally healthy patterns of eating (reduction or elimination of fat, sugar, alcohol, and coffee and an increase in fresh vegetables and fibre), which most people with a normal digestion can tolerate without side effects.

Some diets, such as veganism or macrobiotics, are restrictive and can lead to complications such as reduced bone mass or anaemia, especially in children. Children, pregnant and lactating women, and patients with chronic illness should undertake such major dietary changes with care. A drawback of any dietary change can be social disruption when a patient cannot share meals with friends and family.

High dose nutritional supplementation can lead to acute adverse effects such as diarrhoea (vitamin C) and flushing (niacin) during treatment. Persistent or more serious adverse effects are rare for water-soluble vitamins, although chronic use of high dose vitamin B_6 can lead to neuropathies. Adverse effects, though still uncommon, are more likely to result from high doses of fat-soluble vitamins: vitamin A has been linked with birth defects (if taken during pregnancy) and irreversible bone and liver damage, and vitamin D with hypercalcaemia. High doses of single minerals or amino acids may induce deficiency in nutrients that share similar metabolic pathways. Vitamins and minerals can interfere with chemotherapy and radiotherapy; accordingly, cancer patients are advised to avoid supplements during treatment, and for a few weeks before and after.

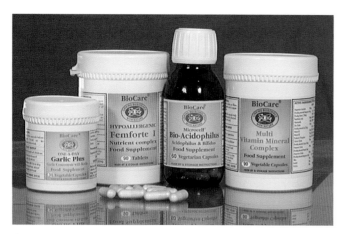

Figure 10.5 Some typical nutritional supplements. Though often perceived by the public to be inherently safe, supplements can sometimes be associated with adverse effects, especially when taken in high doses for long periods.

Practitioners

Decisions to make unconventional nutritional changes are reached by many routes, often through the use of self-help books, leaflets, and magazine articles or advice from friends, relatives, and staff of health food stores. People may also make changes on the basis of nutritional tests provided by commercial companies that advertise laboratory services in the pages of health magazines.

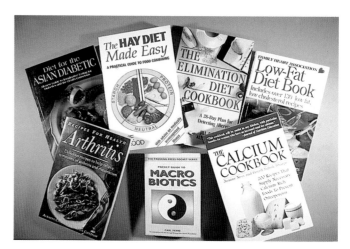

Figure 10.6 Many patients undertake unconventional diets without advice from a practitioner of any kind.

Nutritional consultations may be given by a wide range of practitioners with varying levels of training and experience, from complementary practitioners who mainly practise other disciplines, through trained nutritional therapists and naturopaths, to nurses and doctors who have undertaken further training in nutrition.

Nutritional medicine can be a relatively expensive form of complementary medicine. Diagnostic tests can cost from £15 to over £100 per test, nutritional supplements may cost £10–50 a month, and dietary changes involving organic produce, wholefoods, or preparing juices may also have substantial cost implications.

Training

Various courses in nutritional therapy exist, ranging from short courses of a few days leading to a certificate in basic nutrition, to 3-year, part-time courses leading to qualification as a nutritional therapist. Some courses in nutritional therapy are provided by universities, are underpinned with anatomy and physiology, and lead to the award of a BSc. Naturopaths in Britain usually undergo a 4-year, full-time training, which includes anatomy, physiology, biochemistry, and pathology as well as naturopathic (including nutrition) and osteopathic principles and practice.

The British Society for Allergy, Environmental, and Nutritional Medicine is an association of doctors with a special interest in nutrition. It organizes educational events and publishes the *Journal of Nutritional and Environmental Medicine*.

Regulation

The General Naturopathic Council and the Nutritional Therapy Council are the emerging voluntary, self-regulatory bodies in the

Box 10.5 **Training and educational organizations**

- Department of Nutritional Medicine, University of Surrey: offers part-time postgraduate courses up to MSc level aimed at doctors, dieticians, and nutritional therapists
  c/o Course Administrator for Nutritional Medicine, School of Biological Sciences, University of Surrey, Guildford, Surrey GU2 5XH, UK. Tel: 0148 387 6465; fax: 0148 387 6481; URL: http://www.surrey.ac.uk (access via postgraduate study/taught courses/health and medical sciences)
- Nutrition Matters: an organization offering courses in nutrition for doctors and other biological science graduates
  Redlands, Newbury Park, Ledbury HR8 1AU, UK. Tel: 0168 456 0124; email: info@nutrition-matters.co.uk; URL: http://www.nutrition-matters.co.uk
- British Society for Allergy, Environmental and Nutritional Medicine (BSAENM): membership organization for doctors only
  For publications: PO Box 28, Totton, Southampton SO40 2ZA, UK. Tel: 0238 081 2124
  For enquiries: PO Box 7, Knighton LD7 IWT, UK. Tel: premierline 0906 302 0010

Box 10.6 **Voluntary, self-regulatory bodies for naturopathy and nutrition**

- General Naturopathic Council
  PO Box 73, Okehampton, Devon EX20 1WE, UK. email: info@gncouncil.com; URL: http://www.gncouncil.com
- Nutritional Therapy Council
  PO Box 6114, Bournemouth BH1 9BL, UK. email: info@nutritional-therapycouncil.org.uk; URL: http://www.nutritionaltherapycouncil.org.uk

UK for naturopathy and nutritional therapy. They bring together organizations registering naturopathic practitioners, organizations registering nutritional therapists, and educational establishments providing training, to develop regulatory structures for those professions. Details of the member organizations holding existing registers of practitioners can be found on their websites.

Further reading

Anthony H, Birtwhistle S, Eaton K, Maberly J. *Environmental Medicine in Clinical Practice*. Southampton: BSAENM Publications, 1997.

Brostoff J, Gamlin L. *Complete Guide to Food Allergy and Intolerance*. London: Bloomsbury, 1992.

Davies S, Stewart A. *Nutritional Medicine*. London: Pan, 1987.

Murray M, Pizzorno J. *Encyclopaedia of Natural Medicine*, 2nd edn. London: Prima Publishing, 1997.

Shils M, Olison J, Shike M. *Modern Nutrition in Health and Disease*, 10th edn. London: Lea and Febiger, 2005.

CHAPTER 11

Complementary Medicine and the Patient

Catherine Zollman

The most recent large-scale study of complementary and alternative medicine (CAM) use in the UK estimated that at least 20% of the population had received one CAM therapy from a practitioner. More than half of the respondents using CAM in the past 12 months had not told their general practitioner. In surveys of users of complementary medicine, about 80% are satisfied with the treatment they received. Interestingly, this is not always dependent on an improvement in their presenting complaint. For example, in one UK survey of cancer patients, changes attributed to complementary medicine included being emotionally stronger, less anxious, and more hopeful about the future even if the cancer remained unchanged.

Satisfaction may influence further use of complementary medicine: in one survey over two-thirds of CAM users returned for further courses of treatment and over 90% thought that they might use complementary medicine in the future. What is it that patients find worthwhile and what does this tell us about their expectations of healthcare services in general?

Attractions of complementary medicine

The specific effects of particular therapies obviously account for a proportion of patient satisfaction, but surveys and qualitative research show that many patients also value some of the general attributes of complementary medicine. These may include the relationship with their practitioner, the ways in which illness is explained, and the environment in which they receive treatment. When these augment the therapeutic outcome of treatment, they contribute to what is sometimes called the 'placebo effect'. None of these are unique to complementary medicine, but many are facilitated by the private, non-institutional settings in which most complementary practitioners work. The relative therapeutic importance of specific and non-specific attributes obviously depends on individual patients and practitioners, but some complementary practitioners may be better than their conventional colleagues at using and maximizing the placebo effect.

Time and continuity

Patients often cite the amount of time available for consultation as a reason for choosing complementary medicine, and contrast this with their experiences of seeing conventional NHS doctors. This is partly a feature of all private medicine, but even when

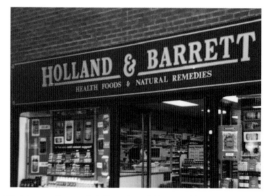

Figure 11.1 Increasing availability of, and demand for, complementary medicine is evidence of its popularity. The question is whether this represents a passing fashion or a deeper need for change within the healthcare system. Reproduced with permission of Holland and Barrett.

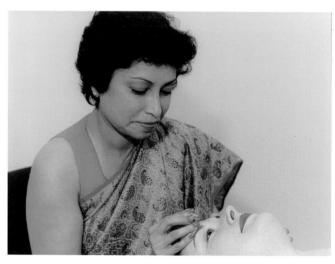

Figure 11.2 Patients seem to appreciate the time and attention they receive during a complementary medicine consultation. Reproduced with permission of the Royal London Homeopathic Hospital.

complementary practitioners work in the NHS their first appointments tend to be up to an hour long in order to take the detailed case history that diagnosis and treatment requires.

When the problem is chronic and multifactorial, in particular, this type of consultation, where patients are encouraged to explain their experience and understanding of their problem, can itself be therapeutic. Patients also generally see the same complementary practitioner over their course of treatment, and this continuity further facilitates the development of a therapeutic patient–practitioner relationship.

Attention to personality and personal experience

All healthcare practitioners, conventional or complementary, aim to tailor their interventions to the needs of individual patients. However, conventional practitioners generally direct treatment at the underlying disease processes, whereas many complementary practitioners base treatment more on the way patients experience and manifest their disease, including their psychology and response to illness. Treatment is 'individualized' in both cases, but patients' personalities and emotions may be more influential in the latter approach.

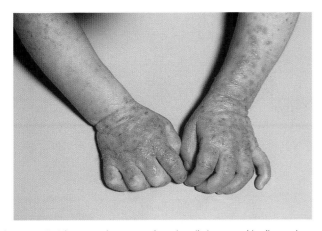

Figure 11.3 Whereas a doctor may be primarily interested in diagnosing atopic dermatitis from other skin conditions, complementary practitioners often take as much account of personality and emotions as they do of physical signs and symptoms. Reproduced with permission of the National Medical Slide Bank.

Although good conventional care involves considering the patient as a person, not a disease, time pressures can lead to an apparent emphasis on the physical aspects of illness. Some patients cite the lack of personal attention paid by conventional practitioners as a reason for choosing a complementary approach. The quality of personal attention is obviously influenced by time and continuity as described above.

Patient involvement and choice

Some users cite the increased opportunities for active participation in the process of recovery as a reason for choosing complementary medicine. Although self-help measures are increasingly part of conventional healthcare advice, patients feel that complementary practitioners give this greater emphasis.

Patients also value being able to choose a complementary therapist or therapy that suits them. To some extent, this is true of all private sector health care, but it is also possible when a choice of different complementary approaches is available on the NHS. An example would be the range of complementary therapies available in many hospices.

Very few evidence-based guidelines are available to support patients in their choice of CAM therapy. Where information has been developed it tends to focus on advising patients about complementary therapies for specific conditions such as cancer. The information provided by NHS Direct is very limited.

Hope

Patients often come to complementary medicine after trying everything that conventional medicine has to offer. Complementary practitioners can offer hope to such patients, both by attempting to influence the underlying disease and, often more importantly, by addressing emotional states, energy levels, coping styles, and other aspects that contribute to quality of life. This is particularly important for patients with chronic diseases and no prospect of cure from conventional medicine. However, practitioners need to balance their claims carefully, considering the realistic chances of improvement and the dangers of creating false hope and further disappointment.

Touch

Many complementary treatments and diagnostic techniques involve more physical contact between patients and practitioners than is usual in conventional medicine. Touch can facilitate more open and honest communication, and patients may turn to the 'low tech' consulting rooms of aromatherapists and reflexologists for a less distancing and more human experience of health care.

Box 11.1 **Attitudes to touch through massage**

- *Staff member in learning difficulties unit* – 'People with profound disabilities often become isolated from any special caring touch. It's inappropriate for us to go around hugging and cuddling pupils, but we can use hand and foot massage'
- *Cancer patient* – 'They're too busy, the nurses, … rushing round the wards … With massage, as soon as the hands go on, you know she's there, she's calm, she's touching you, she has time for you'
- *Patient in primary care* – 'Touch had never been common in my family. Massage has been complementary in giving me a structured experience of touch. The main benefit, though, was relearning to be at ease with my body, relax my mind, without being overcome with weeping or anxieties'

Dealing with ill-defined symptoms

Practitioners of modern Western medicine have become expert in recognizing, identifying, and treating disease. When there is no organic disease present but simply ill-defined symptoms or a general 'lack of health' they may have less to offer. As a result, patients presenting with illnesses such as chronic fatigue, functional back pain, or irritable bowel syndrome may feel that their doctor does not take their symptoms seriously or does not really believe that they are ill. Complementary practitioners do not need a conventional diagnosis to initiate treatment; in fact, many think that their treatments are most effective in patients without organic pathology.

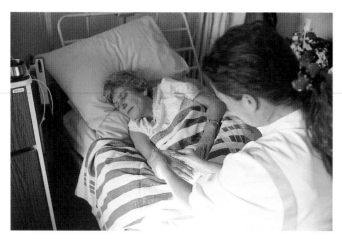

Figure 11.4 Aromatherapy massage in a hospice. Many forms of complementary medicine involve physical contact with patients. Reproduced with permission of John Cole/Impact.

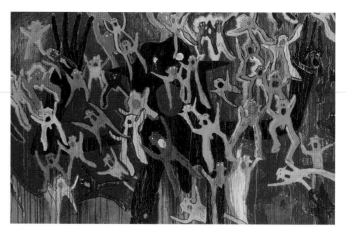

Figure 11.5 *Prostate Roar* by Ian Summers (1998), painted during art therapy after his prostate cancer had been diagnosed. Art therapy, like many other complementary therapies, can help patients to construct a meaningful narrative of disease. Reproduced with permission of the University of Pennsylvania Cancer Center.

Box 11.2 **Example of a complementary practitioner's view of illness**

A patient with chronic ear infections consulted a complementary practitioner, who associated his problem with bad dietary habits and longstanding digestive problems:

   She said that, from a holistic point of view, if you cannot eliminate in the normal way, where does the residual muck go? It can go into your eyes, your breath, and your ears. And, lo and behold, I realised it. She said I was excreting rubbish through my ears, and this, of course, fitted into place, because it was black and sticky. No one ever told me that; they just said, 'You're producing too much wax.'

From Sharma (1995).

Making sense of illness

Patients often want to incorporate their experience of illness into their understanding of themselves and their world. They ask questions like 'Why has this happened to me?' and 'What in my life has caused my problem?' Complementary practitioners may have explanations that make sense to patients – such as describing illness as a result of environmental factors or as a physical expression of emotional patterns.

   Conventional medicine may have problems with such explanations if they have no scientific justification, but sociological research shows that patients consider them beneficial when they reinforce their own beliefs and expectations. Sometimes the explanations given by complementary practitioners can cause problems – for example, if illness is attributed to childhood vaccinations or patients are made to feel guilty for past behaviour.

Spiritual and existential concerns

Some patients have existential concerns that conventionally trained professionals may not feel competent to address. These range from the otherwise healthy adolescent who can find no meaning or purpose in life to the terminally ill patient confronting his or her own mortality. Many complementary disciplines make no distinction between spiritual symptoms and any other types of

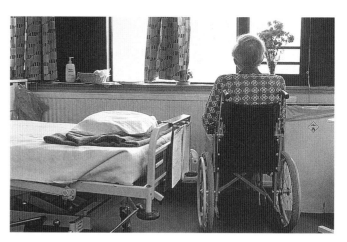

Figure 11.6 Conventional medicine may leave patients' spiritual and existential concerns unmet. Reproduced with permission of Tony Stone Images/Adam Hinton.

symptom and offer treatments aimed at this aspect of a person's life or illness.

Concerns over complementary medicine

The general attributes of complementary medicine do not always lead to increased patient satisfaction. Complementary medicine has some features that can cause patients problems or produce negative effects. Those that primarily involve patients' practical or emotional responses are described below. Those that may pose risks to patients' overall health care are covered in the chapters on individual therapies.

Safety and competence

There is public anxiety that some CAM practitioners may not be adequately qualified, although patients who have already used complementary medicine show less concern. Patients' inability to trust in the competence of their complementary practitioner will influence their experience of treatment. The lack of nationally recognized professional standards for some therapies is a major problem.

Patients often make assumptions about the safety of complementary medication bought over the counter. As many of these contain pharmacologically active agents, they have the potential for adverse effects, particularly where they are taken in combination with other complementary or conventional medication.

Guilt

One potential danger of empowering patients to play an active part in improving their health is that some come to believe that they are solely responsible for their ill health or lack of recovery. For example, patients who are encouraged to take a positive attitude in fighting cancer can suffer increased distress if they infer that their illness is a product of an excessively negative personality. Complementary practitioners need to be aware of this potential when giving advice and explanations to vulnerable patients.

Box 11.3 Potential for inducing guilt and blame in complementary medicine literature

- *Louise Hay* – 'All disease comes from a state of unforgiveness'
- *Edward Bach* – 'Rigidity of mind will give rise to those diseases which produce rigidity and stiffness of the body'
- *Alexander Lowen* – 'A weakness in the backbone must be reflected in serious personality disturbance … the individual with sway back cannot have the ego strength of a person whose back is straight'

Denial

Some patients continue to try different CAM therapies even though none has given any relief. This behaviour can promote an unhelpful pattern of denial about a condition. Repeated attempts to find a cure through complementary medicine can prevent appropriate acceptance and adjustment. Complementary practitioners need to be aware of the risks of colluding with this behaviour.

Blame

Some of the explanations given by complementary practitioners emphasize external and environmental causes of illness. For example, they may claim a disease is caused by vaccinations, conventional drugs, drinking water, dental fillings, or pollution.

Placing the blame for ill health solely on external factors that cannot easily be altered may lead to patients feeling victimized, disempowered, and bitter. There may be other factors influencing their illness, and helpful coping strategies, that could be more usefully addressed.

Financial risk

The amount of money some patients spend on complementary medicine is considerable. Costs vary widely, and higher prices do not necessarily mean better or more effective treatment. The lack of evidence concerning many complementary interventions means that the likelihood of a successful outcome is often impossible to predict. Patients should be aware of this risk. They should also be encouraged to ask practitioners, and seek guidance from the main regulatory bodies, about estimated costs for a complete course of treatment, including tests and medications, before starting complementary therapy.

Box 11.4 Examples of disease-specific sources of information about CAM

- Cancer Backup complementary therapy guide: http://www. cancerbackup.org.uk/Treatments/Complementarytherapies/ Generalinformation/Patientinformationguide
- Arthritis Research Council booklet on complementary therapies: http://www.arc.org.uk/about_arth/booklets/6007/6007.htm
- Multiple Sclerosis Society guide to complementary therapies: http://www.mssociety.org.uk/downloads/ms_essentials_18_complementary_and_alternative_medicine.fc161bb.pdf
- Asthma UK leaflet on non-drug approaches to managing asthma: http://www.asthma.org.uk/all_about_asthma/medicines_treatments/complementary.html

---

Social factors

Most users of complementary medicine in Britain are of middle to high socioeconomic status. Possibly as a result, the effects of poverty, poor housing, and discrimination are underplayed in complementary accounts of disease causation.

Further reading

Benson H. *Timeless Healing; the power and biology of belief.* London: Simon and Schuster, 1996.

Bishop B. *A Time to Heal,* 2nd edn. London: Arkana, 1996.

Sharma U. *Complementary Medicine Today: practitioners and patients,* revised edn. London: Routledge, 1995.

Index